Magnet Environments: Supporting the Retention and Satisfaction of Nurses

Guest Editor

KAREN S. HILL, RN, DNP, NEA-BC, FACHE

NURSING CLINICS OF NORTH AMERICA

www.nursing.theclinics.com

Consulting Editor
SUZANNE S. PREVOST, PhD, RN, COI

March 2011 • Volume 46 • Number 1

SAUNDERS an imprint of ELSEVIER, Inc.

W.B. SAUNDERS COMPANY

A Division of Elsevier Inc.

1600 John F. Kennedy Blvd., Suite 1800 • Philadelphia, PA 19103-2899

http://www.theclinics.com

NURSING CLINICS OF NORTH AMERICA Volume 46, Number 1
March 2011 ISSN 0029-6465, ISBN-13: 978-1-4557-0473-6

Editor: Katie Hartner
Developmental Editor: Donald Mumford

Nursing Clinics of North America (ISSN 0029-6465) is published quarterly by Elsevier Inc., 360 Park Avenue South, New York, NY 10010-1710. Months of issue are March, June, September, and December. Periodicals postage paid at New York, NY and additional mailing offices. Subscription price per year is, $135.00 (US individuals), $343.00 (US institutions), $244.00 (international individuals), $419.00 (international institutions), $197.00 (Canadian individuals), $419.00 (Canadian institutions), $74.00 (US students), and $121.00 (international students). To receive student/resident rate, orders must be accompanied by name of affiliated institution, date of term, and the signature of program/residency coordinator on institution letterhead. Orders will be billed at individual rate until proof of status is received. Foreign air speed delivery is included in all *Clinics* subscription prices. All prices are subject to change without notice. **POSTMASTER:** Send address changes to *Nursing Clinics*, Elsevier Health Sciences Division, Subscription Customer Service, 3251 Riverport Lane, Maryland Heights, MO 63043. **Customer Service: Telephone: 1-800-654-2452** (U.S. and Canada); **1-314-447-8871 (outside U.S. and Canada). Fax: 1-314-447-8029. E-mail: journalscustomerservice-usa@elsevier.com** (for print support) and **journalsonlinesupport-usa@elsevier.com** (for online support).

Nursing Clinics of North America is covered in *EMBASE/Excerpta Medica, MEDLINE/PubMed (Index Medicus), Social Sciences Citation Index, Current Contents, ASCA, Cumulative Index to Nursing, RNdex Top 100,* and Allied Health Literature and International Nursing Index (INI).

Printed and bound by CPI Group (UK) Ltd, Croydon, CR0 4YY

Transferred to Digital Print 2011

Contributors

CONSULTING EDITOR

SUZANNE S. PREVOST, PhD, RN, COI
Associate Dean, Practice and Community Engagement, University of Kentucky, Lexington, Kentucky

GUEST EDITOR

KAREN S. HILL, RN, DNP, NEA-BC, FACHE
Vice President/Nurse Executive, Central Baptist Hospital Administration, Lexington, Kentucky

AUTHORS

KAREN BALAKAS, PhD, RN, CNE
Professor and Director of Clinical Research Partnerships, Goldfarb School of Nursing at Barnes-Jewish College, St Louis, Missouri

JOAN ELLIS BEGLINGER, RN, MSN, MBA, FACHE, FAAN
Vice President for Patient Care Services, St Mary's Hospital, Madison, Wisconsin

TERRY BRYANT, MBA, BSN, RN, NE-BC
Director, Professional Practice and Systems, St Louis Children's Hospital, St Louis, Missouri

DALE CALLICUTT, MSN, RN-BC, CCRN
Staff Development Clinician, Forsyth Medical Center; Adjunct Faculty, Winston-Salem State University, Winston-Salem; Adjunct Faculty, University of North Carolina at Greensboro, Greensboro, North Carolina; Vice Chair, Cardiac-Vascular Nurse Content Expert Panel, ANCC, Silver Spring, Maryland

ELIZABETH CARLSON, PhD, RN
Associate Professor, Department of Adult Health and Gerontological Nursing, Rush University College of Nursing, Chicago, Illinois

PATRICIA S. DAVIS, RN
Project Coordinator, Bassett Medical Center, Cooperstown, New York

PAULA J. DILLON, MS, RN
Director, Department of Medical/Surgical Nursing, Rush University Medical Center, Chicago, Illinois

MARIANNE DITOMASSI, RN, MSN, MBA
Executive Director, Patient Care Services Operations, Massachusetts General Hospital, Boston, Massachusetts

KAREN DRENKARD, PhD, RN, NEA-BC, FAAN
Director, Magnet Recognition Program, American Nurses Credentialing Center,
Sliver Spring, Maryland

JEANETTE IVES ERICKSON, RN, MS, FAAN
Senior Vice President for Patient Care and Chief Nurse, Nursing and Patient Care
Services, Massachusetts General Hospital, Boston, Massachusetts

BRENDA FISCHER, RN, PhD, MBA, CPHQ
Director, Center for Nursing Excellence, Palomar Pomerado Health, San Diego, California

VALENTINA GOKENBACH, RN, DM
Magnet Recognition Program, American Nurses Credentialing Center, Sliver Spring,
Maryland

BARBARA HAUGE, RN, BSN
Unit Director, Medical/Surgical, St Mary's Hospital, Madison, Wisconsin

JEANNE-MARIE HAVENER, PhD, APRN, CNS, FNP
Chair, Department of Nursing, Hartwick College, Oneonta, New York

KAREN S. HILL, RN, DNP, NEA-BC, FACHE
Vice President/Nurse Executive, Central Baptist Hospital Administration, Lexington,
Kentucky

BARBARA HINCH, DNP, RN, ACNP-BC
Assistant Professor, Department of Adult Health and Gerontological Nursing,
Rush University College of Nursing, Chicago, Illinois

PATRICIA JAMERSON, PhD, RN, CRA, CCRP
Nurse Scientist Researcher, Professional Practice and Systems, St Louis Children's
Hospital, St Louis, Missouri

CONNIE JASTREMSKI, MS, MBA, APRN
Chief Nursing Officer, Vice President of Patient Care Services, Bassett Medical Center,
Cooperstown, New York

SHERYL KRAUSE, RN, MS, CEN, ACNS-BC
Clinical Nurse Specialist, Emergency Services, St Mary's Hospital, Madison, Wisconsin

DARIA KRING, PhD, RN-BC
Director of Nursing Research, Forsyth Medical Center, Winston-Salem, North Carolina

JANE LLEWELLYN, PhD, RN, NEA-BC
Vice President, Chief Nursing Officer, and Associate Dean for Practice, Rush University
Medical Center, Chicago, Illinois

PAMELA A. MAXSON-COOPER, MS, BSN, RN, NEA-BC
Nursing Consultant, Froedtert Health, Menomonee Falls, Wisconsin

KAREN L. MAXWELL, MSN, RN-BC
Clinical Nurse Specialist, Saint Joseph's Hospital, Atlanta, Georgia

MARCIA MURPHY, DNP, RN, ANP-BC, FAHA
Assistant Professor, Department of Adult Health and Gerontological Nursing,
Rush University College of Nursing, Chicago, Illinois

MAUREEN FITZGERALD MURRAY, MS, RN, NE-BC
Director, Professional Nursing Practice, Nursing Department, Bassett Medical Center, Cooperstown, New York

KAREN PROFITT NEWMAN, EdD, MSN, RN, NEA-BC
Vice President and Chief Nursing Officer, Department of Administration, Baptist Hospital East, Louisville, Kentucky

AUDREY NICHOLS, RN-BC
Staff Development Clinician, Forsyth Medical Center, Winston-Salem, North Carolina

KAREN NORMAN, MSN, RN-BC, CCRN
Nurse Manager, Forsyth Medical Center; Adjunct Faculty, Winston-Salem State University, Winston-Salem, North Carolina

LORIE K. SHOEMAKER, RN, MSN, DHA, NEA-BC
Chief Nurse Executive, Palomar Pomerado Health, Escondido, California

LESA SMITH, MSN, RN-BC, CCRN
Staff Development Clinician, Forsyth Medical Center; Adjunct Faculty, Winston-Salem State University, Winston-Salem, North Carolina

MARTHA L. TWICHELL, MS, RN, CCRN
Nursing Education, Human Resources Department, Bassett Medical Center, Cooperstown, New York

LAURA ZIEBARTH, RN, MSN
Clinical Nurse Specialist, NICU and Pediatrics, St Mary's Hospital, Madison, Wisconsin

Contents

Not unlike the general population, the population of nurses is aging. This trend is problematic for the nursing workforce in the light of a predicted shortage yet the extent of the effect of the aging population is unknown. What should individuals older than 45 years know to mitigate the effects of aging both physically and professionally? This article describes the magnitude of the aging nursing workforce issue, explores the myths and realities related to the aging process, discusses evidence-based strategies supporting healthy aging and retention of experienced nurses in one Magnet hospital, and introduces recommendations for further study.

This article describes an evidence-informed strategic planning process and framework used by a Magnet-recognized public health system in California. This article includes (1) an overview of the organization and its strategic planning process, (2) the structure created within nursing for collaborative strategic planning and decision making, (3) the strategic planning framework developed based on the organization's balanced scorecard domains and the new Magnet model, and (4) the process undertaken to develop the nursing strategic priorities. Outcomes associated with the structure, process, and key initiatives are discussed throughout the article.

Transition into the workforce for the new graduate nurse is affected by many factors. New graduate nurses can benefit from support provided through participation in the UHC/AACN Residency Program. The retention of even one graduate nurse saves the employing institution up to an estimated $80,000 annually. St Joseph's Hospital has improved the retention of new graduate nurses from approximately 40% to 100% with the addition of the UHC/AACN Residency Program alongside other system changes. Data are being monitored at St Joseph's and on a national level through this multisite collaborative aimed at improving patient care and increasing nurse retention.

In the current health care climate, economic and cultural conditions have created an optimal opportunity to envision a new direction for nursing as a profession. Nurses find themselves at the formative stages of charting this new direction. The articulation of a professional practice model provides a framework for setting this new direction and thus the achievement of exemplary clinical outcomes. In this article, the authors describe the evolution of the professional practice model at the Massachusetts General Hospital and how the model continues to be evaluated and modified over time by the nurses within the system.

Nursing shared governance (NSG) provides a framework for the professionalization of nursing, provides a broader distribution of decision making across the profession, and allocates decisions based on accountability and role expectations. Shared governance defines staff-based decisions, accountability, roles, and ownership of staff in those activities that directly affect nurses' lives and practice. Although NSG is a somewhat ambiguous concept with a vast application, examining it from the perspective of structure, process, and outcomes can more clearly outline a successful strategy for implementation and growth.

In 1980, Froedtert Hospital opened its doors using an innovative registered nurse scheduling model. The hospital has grown to 500 beds, with over 1,600 registered nurses, and continues to use the 7/70 staffing pattern as a core scheduling model. Registered nurses work a straight seven, 10-hour days, and then have 1 week off, or 26 weeks off a year. For professional registered nurses in acute care, the schedule is predictable and consistent for years. This scheduling pattern has resulted in excellent registered nurse satisfaction, increased retention, and consistency in care delivery teams since 1980.

Professional practice models (PPMs) provide the conceptual framework for establishing professional nursing practice. Integrating a PPM requires complex organizational change. One strategy for integrating a PPM is to directly link the PPM with performance expectations to ensure that underlying beliefs are integrated into everyday practice. This article describes the development, implementation, and successful outcomes of a clinical advancement system that was aligned with a PPM.

Professional certification has been linked to positive patient, system, and nurse outcomes. However, certification rates among nurses remain low. Using tenets from employee engagement theory, we designed strategies to fully engage nurses within our nursing division to pursue certification. After 1 year, certification rates more than doubled in our cardiac departments.

To ensure that nursing as a profession is recognized for the value we provide to our organizations, communities, and the world, a consistent level of practice and professionalism will be necessary. Consistency across the profession can be achieved through support of the framework and structures required for the process of attaining Magnet designation. This article is a case study of an organization that on all levels from economic, manpower, quality, and safety has benefited from the Magnet journey.

Nurse recruitment and the retention of a high-quality workforce are challenging issues facing rural hospitals and health centers. The Bassett Healthcare Network has met these challenges by building a supportive framework to develop and support nurses at every level of their professional careers. The organization has partnered with local colleges to help staff nurses further their education. These and other partnership endeavors, such as the organization's clinical ladder and collaborative continuing nursing education opportunities, are helping Bassett sustain and grow the nursing workforce across 8 counties in rural upstate New York and develop stronger ties with academic partners.

Nursing leadership is committed to advancing the profession of nursing through research and evidence-based practice. Partnerships between the hospital and area academic institutions were formed to develop a comprehensive research program that supported active involvement for frontline staff and provide clinical research opportunities for area faculty. Through this collaborative model, the research program has continually expanded and provided clinical research that is making a difference for patients and families. The commitment of this service/academic research partnership is shown by the close involvement of each in future planning for studies and program development. A collaborative partnership is an excellent means to promote clinical research and support nursing excellence.

The progression of five professional nurses from shared governance council chairs to unit director positions and the progression of three nurses from shared governance council chairs to clinical nurse specialist roles in an 18-year period provide compelling evidence of the impact shared governance has provided in the development of future nurse leaders in our organization. The collective wisdom of those who have lived this experience suggests that the opportunities inherent in these clinical nurse leadership roles make this a logical progression, including getting noticed and nudged, developing an understanding of the big picture, developing a results orientation, and substantial skill acquisition.

THE CLINICS ARE NOW AVAILABLE ONLINE!

Access your subscription at:
www.theclinics.com

FORTHCOMING ISSUES

June 2011
Laboratory Competency Care
Diana B. Morwaski, PhD, CNN,
Guest Editor

September 2011
Pain in Education
Stephen D. Krau, PhD, RN, CNE, CT,
Guest Editor

December 2011
Victims of Abuse
Sharon Stahl, PhD, RN, APN,
Guest Editor

RECENT ISSUES

December 2010
Mental Health Across the Lifespan
Patricia B. Howard, PhD, RN, CNAA, FAAN
and Peggy El-Mallakh, PhD, RN,
Guest Editors

September 2010
Palliative Care and End of Life Care
Marianne Matzo, PhD, RN, FAAN
Guest Editor

June 2010
Uniformed Services Nursing
Deborah J. Kenny, PhD, RN
Lieutenant Colonel, US Army (retired),
and Bonnie M. Jennings, DNSc, RN, FAAN,
Colonel, US Army (retired),
Guest Editors

Preface

Magnet Hospitals: Recruiting and Retaining Nurses

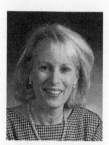

Karen S. Hill, RN, DNP, NEA-BC, FACHE
Guest Editor

It is an honor to serve as the guest editor of this edition of *Nursing Clinics of North America*. The recruitment of talented, dedicated nurses and the retention of these professionals in all realms of nursing practice are essential elements of nurse executive practice. The development and support of structures undergirding workforce development should not be minimized in importance in any organization or practice setting. Successful outcomes in recruitment and retention and thus nurse satisfaction are essential for leaders targeting resource stewardship, standards of excellence, and quality in care delivery. It has been demonstrated that the retention of experienced, skilled nurses supports knowledge transfer between generations of nurses.[1]

Lower vacancy and turnover rates for nursing staff were two outcomes identified among the early research in Magnet organizations in the 1980s.[2] Today Magnet-designated organizations rise to the forefront of innovation and evidence-based leadership in the exploration, investigation, planning, implementation, and evaluation of programs and services to support the recruitment, retention, and satisfaction of the nursing workforce. Research including data from Magnet facilities has identified a significant relationship between experience in nursing and improved patient outcomes.[3] Recruitment and retention have been elevated as key strategies within higher performing organizations.[4] A continuing commitment to innovation was evident when the original call for articles was made for this edition, resulting in more than 58 submitted proposals. The 13 articles that were selected provide a range of perspectives, topics, and expertise from a variety of care settings, all supporting nursing recruitment, retention, and satisfaction. Regardless of the topic, key words including governance, excellence, empowerment, and leadership are common among these articles, again reflecting the principles of a Magnet culture of inclusion and structure. Recruitment

Nurs Clin N Am 46 (2011) xiii–xiv
doi:10.1016/j.cnur.2010.10.012
0029-6465/11/$ – see front matter © 2011 Elsevier Inc. All rights reserved.

and retention are, however, complex issues as is reflected in the diversity of topics presented in this edition.

Nurses in all areas of practice have a responsibility to be informed regarding internal and external forces affecting workforce supply and demand, applications of evidence in leadership leading to "best practice" environments, and the benefits of continuing education competency development as they strategically plan their careers. As professionals, we have a responsibility and accountability for our own career enhancement and job satisfaction; however, organizational culture matters! As is evident in this collection of articles, Magnet hospitals support environments conducive to innovation and success in recruitment and retention.

Karen S. Hill, RN, DNP, NEA-BC, FACHE
Central Baptist Hospital
1740 Nicholasville Road
Lexington, KY 40503, USA

E-mail address:
khill@bhsi.com

REFERENCES

1. Bleich M, Cleary B, Davis K, et al. Mitigating knowledge loss: a strategic imperative for nurse leaders. JONA 2009;39(4):160–4.
2. McClure M, Poulin M, Sovie M, et al. Magnet hospitals: attraction and retention of professional nurses. Kansas City (MO): American Nurses Association; 1983.
3. Clarke S, Aiken L. An international hospital outcomes research agenda focused on nursing: lessons from a decade of collaboration. J Clin Nurs 2008;17:3317–23.
4. Hill K. Improving quality and patient safety by retaining nursing expertise. Online J Issues Nurs 2010;15(3).

Nursing and the Aging Workforce: Myths and Reality, What Do We Really Know?

Karen S. Hill, RN, DNP, NEA-BC, FACHE

KEYWORDS

- Aging • Myths • Healthy aging • Registered nurse • Retirement
- Magnet • Shortage • Stereotypes

NURSING AND THE AGING WORKFORCE: MYTHS AND REALITY

The rapidly growing aging nursing workforce, defined as registered nurses (RNs) older than 45 years, contributes to the predicted shortage of nurses.[1] This article describes the magnitude of the issue of the aging nursing workforce, explores the myths and realities of aging, and presents the evidence-based strategies prevalent in one Magnet environment targeted to address the challenges of aging thus promoting the retention of nurses. Research findings focused on nursing workforce are limited with regard to the issues of aging and the effect of the current age shift on recruitment and retention.

MAGNITUDE OF THE ISSUE: THE AGING NURSING WORKFORCE

Obtaining an accurate calculation of the numbers of nurses older than 45 years is a difficult endeavor; however, it is known that the numbers are growing. Buerhaus and collegues[2] reported that there were 100,000 nurses older than 50 years in 1980 in contrast to more than 400,000 nurses in 2007. In 2008, the average age of an RN in the United States was reported to be 47 years, an increase from 46.8 years reported in 2004.[3] The bigger shift is in the number of RNs older than 50 years, which is 45%, an increase from 33% in 2000.[3] What are the implications of these trends on the nursing workforce? Among other effects including the effect on quality,[4] these figures represent a looming retirement and significant impact within the nursing workforce today.

The general workforce in America is aging, with 20% of the workers expected to be 55 years or older by 2015.[5] From 1998 to 2006, the number of civilian workers, 55 years

The author has nothing to disclose.
Central Baptist Hospital Administration, 1740 Nicholasville Road, Lexington, KY 40503, USA
E-mail address: khill@bhsi.com

and older increased by 49.9%, whereas those aged 25 to 54 years increased by only 5.5%.[5] Life expectancies are increasing. In the report Profile of Older Americans: 2007, it is reported that persons 65 years and older have an average life expectancy of an additional 18.7 years from the previous predictions: 20.0 years for women and 17.1 years for men.[6]

Further, research findings are clear regarding the effect of experience on nursing practice and quality outcomes.[7-9] Uhrenfeldt and Hall[7] described the proficient experienced nurse as making decisions based on ethical discernment and critical observations. In this study, the proficient nurse was reported to have wisdom. Daley[8] relates the development of professional expertise to the transition from serial problem solving to stages of career development. The perspectives and actions of nurses are affected by levels of experience. Novice nurses identify issues such as time management or lack of educational preparation as constraints to quality practice. Experienced nurses report barriers in more of a systems approach, such as the method in which assignments are made or the levels of support systems available to aid them in performing their role. Taylor[9] cites an example of the dichotomy between novice and expert perspective by suggesting that the inability to recognize meaningful information and relate to possible causal factors is influenced by a combination of lack of clinical expertise and stress. Professional experience, nursing expertise in the provision of clinical care, and a maturity of perspective and critical thinking hold advantages for the patient and the health care system in ensuring quality outcomes.

Awareness of the predicted large scale exodus of aging nurses from the workforce has spurred some creativity in approaches to retention. Phased retirement has been suggested as one solution to bridge the knowledge gap between novice and expert practices and has been widely implemented in academic organizations.[10] Hospitals and employers of nurses have been slower to adopt this innovative approach to retention. In a recent survey, only 7% of the surveyed hospitals (N = 41) reported any type of phased retirement plan and only 9% reported formal succession planning initiatives even though both programs are proposed solutions for preserving clinical knowledge and expertise.[11] There is a paucity of research data to support whether phased retirement is an effective strategy to retain expertise within the nursing profession. It is clear, nonetheless, that the aging of the population of nurses and thus the nursing workforce is not a myth but a reality and that the retention of expertise within nursing has an effect on patient outcomes and nursing practice and must be strategically addressed.

Thornton[12(p311)] summarized the science around the issue of the aging population by concluding that "considering the aging population issues that need to be addressed in the next four decades, developmental and longitudinal studies of individuals and cohorts after middle age are extremely sparse and are a priority." Perceptions of successful aging are multidimensional and include physical, mental, and social parameters.[13] Addressing the myths of aging with data and education is a way to increase opportunities for older nurses within the workforce and maximize the benefits of knowledge and expertise for the patient.

MYTHS ASSOCIATED WITH AGING
Physical Abilities

Myths, defined as "a widely held mistaken belief,"[14] are often focused on negative images and stereotypes. Research about aging has predominately reported dismal predictions of functional declines in both physical and mental capacities. The concepts of healthy or successful aging are beginning to counteract the negative images of growing old.[13] However, the physiologic changes associated with aging have implications for individual worker performance and productivity.[10] Dispelling myths surrounding those changes with data is essential to maximize career opportunities for the older worker and outcomes for the system. The following are some of the most common myths of aging.

Changes in the physical condition of the older person including deterioration of sensation are inevitable and affect performance

Changes in visual acuity including the need for increased lighting, age-related hearing loss, decreases in musculoskeletal strength, and reduction in joint mobility and manual dexterity are reported as a result of aging.[10] Physical changes associated with aging include decreased bone density, visual acuity, metabolic rate, cardiac function, and respiratory capacity.[15] No research has identified a stage of progression in physical decline related to specific ages. In reality, levels of decline and stamina seem to have a high level of variability.[16] Aging as a continuum moves from independence, to interdependence, and then dependence. It was suggested that a person might be chronologically young and functionally old because the aging process rate may vary significantly related to physical and mental capabilities.[17] Findings demonstrate that individuals older than 65 years at present have fewer physical changes affecting competency in daily physical performance than earlier generations of the same chronologic age.[18] Advances in physical health and stamina are attributed to improvements in medical care, improved economic status of older adults supporting healthier lifestyles, and improved technology to mitigate physical decline.

Higher incidence of workplace injuries are reported for older workers

McMahan and Sturz[10] reported that older workers have a higher risk of workplace injuries. Data indicate that injured older workers sustain disabling injuries more frequently than younger workers.[10] Older workers, however, are less likely to develop disabling conditions from these injuries than younger workers and thus have fewer work days lost and lower cost per injury than younger workers.[10] Strategies to decrease the incidence of injury in older workers includes the use of antislip work surfaces and shoes, the addition of ergonomically designed desks and office furniture, the provision of support for the implementation of devices, such as overhead ceiling lifts, and the development of tailored educational programs related to injury prevention to raise the awareness of safety of older workers.[1,10]

Cognitive Abilities

There are also many myths regarding the deterioration of cognitive abilities of the older worker.

Older people do not want to or cannot learn new skills

In reality, maintaining a high level of everyday intelligence and mental stimulation through work interactions can promote stability in the levels of mental cognition beyond the age of 70 years.[16,18] Memory training programs have also been shown to be effective in individuals younger than 85 years.[18] In a convenience sample of persons older than 50 years,[15] 93% of the respondents reported enjoying learning new skills and acquiring new knowledge, 79% reported an interest in increasing computer skills and obtaining technology-related training, and 77% expressed an interest in receiving updated education related to their vocation. Many older individuals, in fact, display a lifelong commitment to learning.[16] Evidence supports no decrease in the ability of older workers to use accumulated knowledge and word skills.[17]

People have a lack of control over the process of aging
Another myth associated with older workers is that aging people lack control over mental and physical deterioration. Thornton[12(p304)] reported that "while aging cannot be stopped nor reversed, a great deal can be done to influence how individuals experience aging". In reality, the cognitive effects of aging can be mitigated or delayed through the concepts of healthy aging, including diet modification, regular exercise, limits on alcohol consumption, and opportunities for social interaction with others.[12,19] Personality and character traits were reported as heavily influencing a perception of successful aging.[13,16]

Financial Security

Myths abound about the financial security of older individuals.

Getting older equates to negative changes in social and economic status
The strongest predictor of healthy aging was the presence of a social network as defined by close friends, a spouse, or a confidant, although the causality and linkage of specific behaviors to the stages of healthy aging was unclear.[10,16,20] Employment situations often provide large social networks supporting personal and professional interactions as well as financial security.[10,21] Many of the policies and benefit structures in traditional employment arrangements were developed when life expectancy did not extend to the current predicted rates. Vladeck[22] reported that a large number of older Americans are asset rich and cash poor. The decrease in the pool of younger workers and increase in the number of older people contributes to a smaller pool of money for a larger number of retired persons. The increasing financial insecurity during recent times, including rising unemployment, should be further explored for effect on the financial health of older citizens, both working and retired. Turner[23] reported that the labor market for individual workers changes dramatically as they age, affecting the strength of bargaining and leverage that continually takes place between employers and workers. Reinforcing the previous reference to the multidimensional effect of aging, Basta and colleagues.[24] identified that community level socioeconomic status was a strong predictor of cognitive and functional impairment in a selected older population. In a cross-sectional analysis of data, Basta and colleagues.[24] found that individuals living in more deprived areas with lower income potential had a higher prevalence of memory loss and other symptoms of cognition impairment. Improving financial and community resources for older adults including providing opportunities for employment are suggestions to slow the progress of economic decline and increase the probability of financial security.[10,24,25]

GAPS IN THE LITERATURE

Gaps in the literature regarding the aging nursing workforce include further exploration regarding the myths of aging and their relationship to perceptions, stereotypes, and career opportunities within the workplace. Assumptions about the process of aging are often made based on studies of the general workforce formed over many years. Recent advances have taken place in the understanding of health and lifestyle behaviors, which will affect the process of aging, the perception regarding growing older, and career goals and attitudes.

The predominance of women within the nursing workforce leads to a need for further study regarding the effect of gender on aging among older workers because the division between the sexes is atypical of the general population: 49% women in general population versus 93% women in nursing.[26] Longitudinal studies of nursing as a cohort should include monitoring the effect of the physical labor of nursing in comparison to the recommendations for physical activity to support healthy aging. Another gap involves analysis of the progression of physical decline relative to increasing age. Mitigating factors such as diet and exercise need to be studied to support the development of guidelines for nurses as they prepare for aging in the best way possible and therefore remain active in the workforce.

Identification of the presence and type of workplace accommodations to mitigate cognition and sensory changes in the elderly is an important area for further investigation. The Wisdom at Work[1] initiative funded by the Robert Woods Johnson Foundation, provided research and funding for the exploration of interventions to support retention of older nurses. Most accommodations in the piloted interventions focused on the ergonomic components of practice and not the human resource/benefit area. The projects included overhead lift devices, lift teams, redesigned units, ergonomically correct chairs, computer stations, and communication systems; however; few identified nonergonomic accommodations as a solution.[27]

The identification of accommodations based on evidence is an important strategy for the retention of staff and supports an increase in employee productivity and safety with aging workers. Head and colleagues[28] reported on the findings of the Society of Human Resource Management survey of 61 companies. Based on the exploration of a low (3.2%) response rate, it was found that strategies are sparse regarding current practices in the workplace to accommodate older workers and little is known about what to do. It is important to note that the 2 most frequently cited reasons for the lack of participation in the study and the reported low response rate resulted from an inability to delineate specific accommodations for older workers and an inability to identify anyone knowledgeable about these accommodations to complete the survey. In providing further information, company representatives thought that accommodations were being made everyday yet specific examples were not readily available. The feedback from nonparticipants led the researchers to conclude that developing reporting systems to collect workplace data on accommodations for the older worker was of vital importance for the retention and success of older workers, including creating a proactive approach to this growing national dilemma through building a knowledge database.

Other gaps in the literature include the identification of the role of education, with managers both in heightening awareness regarding the benefits of the retention of older employees and in addressing issues of culture and environment to better maximize the usefulness, productivity, and contribution of the older worker. Training and education will reduce stereotypes of ageism among health care professionals.[25] In reality, chronologic age is a weak predictor of capacity for productive performance and contribution,[10] particularly among older nurses, with career opportunities and increasing flexibility.

Predictors of early retirement within the nursing workforce and intent to leave the profession of nursing should be explored within the context of the changing labor market. Poor self-rated health among 5538 Danish nurses[29] is cited as a predictor of early retirement. However, this factor could be a self-perpetuating cycle because the lifestyle typically associated with retirement may contribute to lower physical and health activities. Findings suggest that a physically stressful work environment could cause poor health and thus increase the probability of early retirement.[29] Solutions including scheduling flexibility, improving relationships with supervisors, and the development of programs of phased retirement need to be evaluated within various care settings regarding the effect on work satisfaction and intent to stay in the nursing profession. Among the aging workers surveyed,[30] 93% reported a desire to work in some capacity as they age to supplement their income. What can be done to keep the aging nurses working within the health care industry?

PROPOSED SOLUTIONS FROM ONE MAGNET ORGANIZATION

The Central Baptist Hospital (CBH) in Lexington, KY, USA, a 371-bed acute care facility, received the Magnet designation in 2005 and was redesignated in 2010. Currently, of the almost 1000 RNs on staff, 34% are older than 45 years, the percentage increasing significantly from the 2002 figures of 20%. At the initiation of the Magnet journey, a commitment to age diversity was identified as a strategic priority by nursing and human resource leaders. The following initiatives were implemented at CBH to support the retention of nurses 45 years of age and older.

Development of a Senior Nurse Advisory Council

The Senior Nurse Advisory Council (SNAC) is a group for any RN aged 45 years or older and meets at least twice a year, with 30 minutes of the meeting devoted to socialization and networking and 30 minutes for a presentation of interest to the staff. Topics have included education in personal and retirement finance, open discussions about ideas to improve the working environment at CBH for older nurses, and a presentation about a proposed construction project to solicit input from participants. A benefit realized because of this program has been an increased sense of identity and worth voiced by senior nurses within the organization. Opportunities for social networking have been rated as important on employee engagement surveys by this segment of the workforce, and the SNAC group is one way to support this goal. As noted in **Table 1**, there has been a positive shift in the score of the question "I feel I am a part of a team" from 53% in 2006 to the current score of 90% among RNs aged 46 years and older.

Stratification of Employee Engagement Data

Employee engagement data were stratified to highlight issues of importance to the nurses older than 46 years as depicted in **Table 1**. Data from this analysis have been used to develop human resource plans for RN retention according to career phases and to support the business case for the development of employee wellness programs targeted toward older individuals. In addition, educational programs within the leadership development curriculum have been offered to support communication and management of multigenerational employees. These programs have enabled leaders to openly discuss myths and stereotypes of aging, including their own, in a learning situation and develop strategies to address these myths and stereotypes.

Table 1
Employee engagement survey results

	2010 (% Agree)	2008 (% Agree)	2006 (% Agree)	Health Care Norm 2010 (%)
Overall Satisfaction With CBH as a Place to Work				
RNs 30 y or Younger	89	80	76	79
RNs 46 y or Older	88	74	65	79
I Rarely Think About Looking for Another Job With a New Company				
RNs 30 y or Younger	75	47	55	64
RNs 46 y or Older	86	67	65	64
I Feel I am a Part of a Team				
RNs 30 y or Younger	95	74	73	78
RNs 46 y or Older	90	67	53	78

Implementation of an Innovative Career-Coaching Model

The career coaching program was initially funded through the American Organization of Nurse Executives Foundation as a nursing research project in 2008. The proposal targeted mid- and late-career nurses to provide support for career transition, continuing education, and changes in areas of practice with an ultimate goal to retain these nurses in the workforce and the organization. Employee engagement data supporting outcomes in this area are also summarized in **Table 1**. Results include a dramatic increase in overall workplace satisfaction for RNs older than 46 years from 65% in 2006 to 88% in 2010.

Other initiatives within the organization targeted at workforce enhancement including a new graduate residency program, an evidence-based leadership development program, and the increased support resources for nursing-led projects have also contributed to the positive shifts in employee engagement in both RNs older than 46 years and RNs aged 30 years and younger as well as all in RNs in aggregate.

SUMMARY

Recent changes in retirement patterns suggest that nurses have a willingness to work longer than they anticipated to within the profession and have modified their visions of the "final" stages of their careers.[31] The imperative is now on the employers and society to recognize the value and contributions of the older employee, diminish myths with facts, and implement initiatives to enhance the work environment for the aging nurse thus ensuring retention of senior employees. Recognition of the value of experiential knowledge and expertise benefiting the patients as well as support for economic security and career satisfaction among these employees is key to the quality of care provided.[4] The culture within a Magnet organization is well suited to support innovation regarding dispelling myths of aging and recruitment of seasoned and experienced nurses. Older workers are valuable members of teams in relationship-centered professions such as nursing.[1] Using data to dispel the myths of aging, planning workforce accommodations based on research and accurate projections, and raising the awareness of employers regarding the benefit of retention of older workers, particularly experienced nurses, requires immediate action if the benefit for the system, patient, and nurse are to be maximized.

ACKNOWLEDGMENTS

The author would like to thank Patricia K. Howard, RN, FAAN, Brenda Cleary, RN, FAAN, Karen Stefaniak, RN, and Dorothy Brockopp, RN for their assistance and support with this article.

REFERENCES

1. Hatcher B, Bleich M, Connolley C, et al. Wisdom at work. 2006. Available at: www.rwjf.org/newsroom/newsreleasesdetail.jsp?productid=21894. Accessed August 10, 2008.
2. Buerhaus P, Donelan K, Ulrich B, et al. Trends in the experiences of hospital-employed registered nurses: results from three national surveys. Nurs Econ 2007; 25(2):69–80.
3. Health Resources and Services Administration. 2008 National sample of RNs. 2010. Available at: http://bhpr.hrsa.gov/healthworkforce/rnsurvey/. Accessed August 9, 2010.

4. Hill K. "Improving quality and patient safety by retaining nursing expertise". On-line J Issues Nurs 2010;15(3). Available at: http://www.nursingworld.org/MainMenuCategories/ANAMarketplace/ANAPeriodicals/OJIN/TableofContents/Vol152010/No3-Sept-2010/Articles-Previously-Topic/Improving-Quality-and-Patient-Safety-.aspx. Accessed August 9, 2010.

5. AARP Public Policy Institute. Update on the aged 55+ worker. Data digest No. 136. Washington, DC: AARP Public Policy Institute; 2006. Available at: http://assets.aarp.org/rgcenter/econ/dd136_worker.pdf. Accessed October 28, 2010.

6. U.S. Administration on Aging. Profile of older Americans: 2007. Washington, DC: Administration on Aging; 2007.

7. Uhrenfeldt L, Hall E. Clinical wisdom among proficient nurses. Nurs Ethics 2007; 14(3):387–98.

8. Daley B. Novice to expert: an exploration of how professionals learn. Adult Education Quarterly 1999;49(4):1–17.

9. Taylor C. Assessing patient's needs: does the same information guide expert and novice nurses? Int Nurs Rev 2002;49(1):11–9.

10. McMahan S, Sturz D. Implications for an aging workforce. J Edu Bus 2006;82(1): 50–5.

11. Bleich M, Cleary B, Davis K, et al. Mitigating knowledge loss; "a strategic imperative for nurse leaders". JONA 2009;39(4):160–4.

12. Thornton J. Myths of aging or ageist stereotypes. Educ Gerontol 2002;28:301–12.

13. Phelan E, Anderson L, LaCroix A, et al. Older adults' views of "successful aging"- how do they compare with researchers' definitions? J Am Geriatr Soc 2004;52:211–6.

14. Encarta Dictionary. 2010. Available at: http://encarta.msn.com/encnet/features/dictionary/dictionaryhome.aspx/. Accessed February 14, 2010.

15. Women Ageing and Health: A Framework for Action. (2007). World Health Organization. Available at: C\\...Women-ageing-health-loweres.pdf. Accessed 10/12/2008.

16. Knight T, Ricciardelli L. Successful aging: perceptions of adults aged between 70 and 101 years. Int J Aging Hum Dev 2003;56(3):223–45.

17. Munnell A, Sass S, Soto M. Employer attitudes towards older workers: survey results. Work opportunities for older Americans. Boston (MA): Center for Retirement Research at Boston College; 2006. Series 3, June.

18. Baltes P. New frontiers in the future of aging: from successful aging of the young old to the dilemmas of the fourth age. Gerontology 2003;49(2):123–35.

19. Rowe JW, Kahn RN. Human aging: usual and successful aging. Science 1987; 237:143–9.

20. Michael Y, Colditz G, Coakley E, et al. Health behaviors, social networks, and healthy aging: cross-sectional evidence from nurse's health study. Qual Life Res 1999;8:711–22.

21. Bryant L, Corbet K, Kutner J. In their own words: a model of healthy aging. Soc Sci Med 2001;53(7):927–41.

22. Vladeck BC. Economic and policy implications of improving longevity. J Am Geriatr Soc 2005;53(Suppl 9):304–7.

23. Turner J. Work options for older Americans. Benefits Q, Third Quarter 2008;24(3): 20–5.

24. Basta N, Matthews F, Chatfield M, et al. Community-level socio-economic status and cognitive and functional impairment in the older population. Eur J Public Health 2008;18(1):48–54.

25. Leggett D. The aging work force- helping employees navigate midlife. AAOHN J 2007;55(4):169–75.

26. Buerhaus P, Staiger D, Auerbach D. The future of the nursing workforce in the United States; data, trends and implications. Studbury (MA): Jones & Bartlett; 2008.
27. Hill K, Cleary B, Hewlett P, et al. Commentary: experienced RN retention strategies: what can be learned from top-performing organizations. JONA, in press.
28. Head L, Baker P, Bagwell B, et al. Barriers to evidence-based practice in accommodations for an aging workforce. Work 2006;27(4):391–6.
29. Friis K, Ekholm O, Hundrup E, et al. Influence of health, lifestyle, working conditions and sociodemography on early retirement among nurses: the Danish nurses cohort study. Scand J Public Health 2006;35:23–30.
30. Flores-Reed L. The real talent debate: will aging boomers deplete the workforce? A WorldatWork research report. 2007. Available at: www.worldatwork.org/. Accessed January 29, 2010.
31. Palumbo M, McIntosh B, Rambur B, et al. Retaining an aging nurse workforce: perceptions of human resource practices. Nurs Econ 2009;27(4):221–7.

Creating a Nursing Strategic Planning Framework Based on Evidence

Lorie K. Shoemaker, RN, MSN, DHA, NEA-BC[a],*,
Brenda Fischer, RN, PhD, MBA, CPHQ[b]

KEYWORDS

- Strategic planning • Evidence-based framework
- Magnet • PPH

Somehow there are organizations that effectively manage change, continuously adapting their bureaucracies, strategies, systems, products, services, and cultures to survive the shocks and prosper from the forces that decimate others...they are the masters of what I call renewal.
Robert H. Waterman, Jr—The Renewal Factor.[1]

The twentieth century was ruthless and unforgiving for many industries, including aerospace, airline, banking, and defense. Downsizing, mergers, acquisitions, and closures plagued the United States during that time span. Unfortunately, this trend has continued into the twenty-first century, with the health care industry very much a part of the concomitant chaos. Both public and private health care organizations continue to face a turbulent, a confusing, and an often-threatening environment.[1] The imposed economic constraints of various payor mechanisms, health care legislative and policy initiatives, as well as changing population demographics and advancing technology compel health care organizations to critically analyze their systems and develop strategies aimed at enhancing quality, improving care delivery and service, controlling costs, and increasing market share. According to Swayne and colleagues,[1] positioning an organization to more effectively respond to this changing environment requires focused strategic thinking and planning on the part of the management team as they seek to become "masters of renewal" in this dynamic environment.

Funding support: None.
Financial disclosure: The authors have nothing to disclose.
[a] Palomar Pomerado Health, Nursing Administration, 456 East Grand Avenue, Escondido, CA 92025, USA
[b] Palomar Pomerado Health, Center for Nursing Excellence, 15255 Innovation Drive, San Diego, CA 92128, USA
* Corresponding author.
E-mail address: Lorie.Shoemaker@pph.org

This article describes an evidence-informed strategic planning process and framework used by a California public health care system, representing the full continuum of care on its 5-year strategic planning journey to Magnet Recognition status, involving nurses at all levels of the organization. This article includes (1) an overview of the organization and its strategic planning process, (2) the structure created within nursing for collaborative strategic planning and decision making, (3) the strategic planning framework developed based on the organization's balanced scorecard (BSC) domains and the new Magnet model, (4) the process undertaken to develop the nursing strategic priorities, and (5) the process undertaken for continuous renewal of the strategic planning process. Outcomes associated with the structure, process, and key initiatives are discussed throughout the article.

ORGANIZATIONAL PROFILE

Palomar Pomerado Health (PPH), located in North San Diego County, is the largest public health care district in the state of California, serving an area of 850 square miles encompassing 7 different communities. The health district was founded in 1937 by a registered nurse (RN) and a dietician, who opened a small medical facility on a former poultry farm. Today, the health system comprises the Palomar Medical Center, a 317-bed tertiary medical center and level II trauma center in Escondido, California; the Pomerado Hospital, a 107-bed community hospital in Poway, California; 2 distinct part skilled nursing facilities; a home care division; an ambulatory surgery center; an outpatient behavioral medicine center; a recently opened outpatient women's pavilion; and 2 retail health clinics.

PPH is governed by a 7-membered publicly elected board of directors (BOD), each serving a 4-year term. One chief executive officer oversees the entire health system along with 13 senior level executives who lead the organization and provide a fiscal oversight for its $1.7 billion operating budget. Two-thirds of PPH's 3800 employees are organized for the purposes of collective bargaining. The California Nurses Association is the recognized bargaining agent for the RNs, and the Caregivers Healthcare Employees Union is the bargaining agent for the service and technical employees. Because PPH is a public entity, all BOD proceedings are open to the public, and all, but very few, documents are made available to the public on request. This level of transparency subjects PPH to frequent public and media scrutiny and presents a unique challenge in the strategic planning process.

Directional Strategies

Swayne and colleagues[1] define directional strategies as the organization's mission, vision, and values. The mission should describe the organization's distinctive purpose, the vision as the hope for its future, and the values as the guiding principles that are held dear by its members.

Mission

PPH leadership believes that its role as the largest public health care district in the state imposes a special level of accountability to the community. This is reflected in the PPH mission: "To heal, comfort and promote health in the communities we serve." This mission is a broadly defined enduring statement of the purpose that distinguishes PPH from other organizations and places nursing at the core of the organization's existence.

Vision

In conjunction with a leadership change in 2003, PPH undertook a comprehensive process to craft a new vision, resulting in the aspiration, "Palomar Pomerado Health will be the health system of choice for patients, physicians, and employees, recognized nationally for the highest quality of clinical care and access to comprehensive services." Because the nursing division represents more than 40% of the employees in the organization, the chief nurse executive (CNE) and nurses at all levels were involved in the development of this vision. Attaining the vision is heavily dependent on the quality of nursing services.

Values

The values of PPH were reaffirmed during the drafting of the vision and include the following:

- Compassion—treat patients and their families with dignity, respect, and empathy at all times. Be considerate and respectful to colleagues.
- Integrity—be honest and ethical in all we do, regardless of consequences.
- Teamwork—work together toward a common goal while valuing our differences.
- Innovation and creativity—courageously seek and accept new challenges; take risks.
- Excellence—continuously strive to meet the highest standards to surpass all customer expectations.
- Stewardship—inspire commitment, accountability, and sense of common ownership.

These values are a clear depiction of expected behaviors, beliefs, ideals, and social responsibility and are firmly embedded in the culture of the organization, including the nursing division.

Philosophy and model of care

To achieve the mission and vision, PPH has embraced a philosophy of partnering for excellence, that is, working collaboratively with physicians, staff, vendors, and the community to improve programs and services. The philosophy of nursing services supports and reflects the PPH mission, vision, values, and philosophy by empowering nursing staff to partner with patients and their families, physicians, and other members of the health care team in the provision of excellence in patient care. The tenets of the nursing philosophy are based on the relationship-based care model[2] that is composed of 3 crucial relationships:

1. The care provider's relationship with patient and family
2. The care provider's relationship with self
3. The care provider's relationship with colleagues.

The elements of the relationship-based care model closely align with the 6 core values of PPH, as shown in **Table 1**.

PPH Nursing Vision

Although the nursing division has long embraced the PPH mission, vision, and values, a clear vision for nursing services was lacking when the system CNE assumed her position in 2004. To mitigate this, the CNE embarked on a 6-month journey from August 2004, to February 2005, to meet with as many nursing staff members as possible in one-on-one sessions to get their input into issues of importance to

Table 1	
Crosswalk of PPH values with the relationship-based care model	
PPH Values	**Relationship-Based Care Model**
Compassion	Professional nursing: professional nursing exists to provide compassionate care to individuals and their loved ones. Nursing is a primary component in a complex interdependent health care delivery system.
Integrity	Leadership: leaders know the vision, act with purpose, remove barriers, and consistently hold patients, families, and staff as their priority.
Teamwork	Teamwork requires a group of diverse members from all disciplines and departments to define and embrace a shared purpose and work together to fulfill that purpose.
Innovation and Creativity	Care delivery: The patient care delivery system is the infrastructure for organizing and providing care to patient and families. The system determines the way the activities of care are accomplished and is built on the concepts and values of professional nursing practice.
Excellence	Outcomes: achieving quality outcomes requires planning, precision, and perseverance. It begins with defining specific, attainable, and measurable outcomes.
Stewardship	Resources: a resource-driven practice is one that maximizes all available resources such as staff, time, equipment, systems, and budget.

them. More than 350 nurses at all levels of the organization, across all campuses and shifts, were interviewed. The following are summaries from these meetings:

- Overwhelmingly, the "best thing" about working at PPH was the compassionate caring coworkers and teamwork.
- The nursing staff was pleased with the responsiveness of their managers and supervisors and had many positive comments to share in that regard.
- Most of the staff planned on working at PPH in a patient care setting for 3 to 5 years, with many desiring to further their education and/or achieve certification in their field.
- Staff education, recruitment and retention, and quality patient care were identified as the areas that should be the focus and priority of the organization.

Based on these meetings, a vision and 4-year strategic plan for nursing were developed. The nursing vision is clearly aligned with the overall vision of the organization and specifies, "Palomar Pomerado Health Nursing will be nationally recognized for setting the standard in nursing service excellence in practice, education, research, and leadership. Our nurses are the key." With this vision in mind, the nursing leadership made the decision to use the 14 Forces of Magnetism as the road map to achieve nursing excellence at PPH.

PPH Strategic Planning Process

In 2004, PPH modified its planning process to increase its focus and continuity of strategic goals over a multiyear period. Having crafted a new vision, the executive management team (EMT) wanted to inspire the organization to dream big while also moving dreams toward reality—in a time frame that allowed for realistic incremental improvement. Based on the philosophy that its purpose is to serve patients and the community by providing high-quality patient care that will result in satisfied customers, which in turn will increase market share and financial resources to reinvest in its mission, the EMT identified 4 domains in which the organization must excel:

- Workforce/Workplace development: the human and facilities infrastructure to provide services.
- Quality: high-quality outcomes achieved through the application of evidence-based protocols and safe, efficient, and effective processes.
- Customer service: developing loyal patients and physicians by exceeding their expectations.
- Financial strength: earnings sufficient to fund ongoing operations and growth in services and facilities.

This philosophy and these domains are valid at all levels in the organization and form the basis for the nursing strategic plan. Annually, the BOD, EMT, and department directors hold a strategic planning session to assess progress on annual initiatives and objectives and to develop new initiatives for the coming fiscal year aimed at moving the organization closer to the achievement of the multiyear goals. After approval of the organization's annual strategic initiatives by the BOD, the nursing strategic plan is reviewed and updated with input from nursing staff at all levels. Once finalized, the nursing strategic plan is presented for approval to the 2 decision-making bodies within the nursing division, the Clinical Leadership Council (CLC) and the Professional Practice Council (PPC) (both are defined later in this article). On approval, the individual nursing departments develop initiatives with input from staff and this input further supports the nursing and organizational strategic plan.

The nursing strategic plan encompasses all nursing areas within the health system and is clearly linked to the 4 domains, the long-term goals of the organization, as well as the Forces of Magnetism. **Table 2** outlines select linkages between the PPH long-range goals and objectives and the long-term objectives and initiatives of the nursing division that were adopted in 2005 after the one-on-one interviews with the nursing staff.

Balanced Scorecard

PPH uses a BSC to focus its efforts on activities that are strategically important, to align its efforts across departments and along the continuum of care, and to systematically gather data that support learning and continuous improvement.[3] The scorecard structure reflects the PPH planning and performance management model (**Fig. 1**). BSC is an online tool wherein the goals and initiatives are tracked and monitored at the organizational, divisional, and departmental level and to which staff at all levels of the organization have access to view. Progress on the nursing strategic initiatives is reported monthly to the CLC and PPC. Departmental goals are reviewed at staff meetings and/or Unit Practice Councils, which are run by point-of-care nurses for the purpose of continuous improvement in patient care and professional practice.

Key Nursing Strategic Initiatives and Outcomes

When the original nursing strategic plan was being developed, California was facing the worst nursing shortage in the country with 5.75 RNs per 1000 residents. The nursing shortage in PPH's surrounding area was even worse, with 3.56 RNs per 1000 residents. This shortage led to the creation of 2 key nursing strategic initiatives. One initiative under the financial strength domain was to develop, gain approval, and implement a nursing recruitment strategic plan, and another under the workforce development domain was to develop collaborative relationships

Table 2
Linkage of PPH long-range goals and objectives with nursing objectives and initiatives

PPH Domain	Long-Range Goals	Objective	Nursing Objective	Nursing Initiative
Financial Strength	Achieve Moody Aa bond rating	Achieve profitability	Optimize resource utilization in the delivery of patient care	Develop, gain approval, and implement the nursing recruitment strategic plan
Customer Service	Achieve 90th percentile for physician and patient loyalty	Develop loyal patients	Develop loyal patients	Develop loyal patients through continuous performance improvement of the nursing-sensitive indicators
Quality	Achieve national recognition for clinical quality and performance excellence, including achieving the California Baldrige Award and Magnet Recognition status	Demonstrate high-quality and safe patient care	Achieve recognitions of distinction including ANCC Magnet Recognition status	Achieve national recognition for clinical quality and performance excellence
Workforce/Workplace Development	Achieve national recognition as one of the top health systems in the country to work for, achieve national recognition for development of state-of-the-art facilities and technology	Attract, acquire, and retain a high-quality workforce	Secure optimal nursing personnel to meet the health care needs of the community	Develop collaborative relationships, with the community focused on increasing the supply of well-educated health care professionals

Abbreviation: ANCC, American Nurses Credentialing Center.

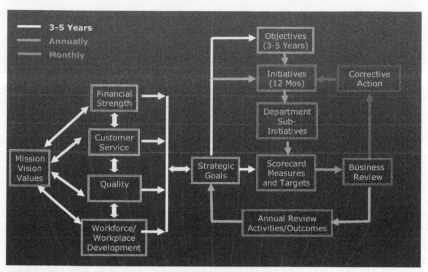

Fig. 1. Planning and business performance management model.

with the community, focused on increasing the supply of well-educated health care professionals (see **Table 2**). To realize the goals of these initiatives, the CNE and PPH Board worked with local colleges and universities to provide funding for additional faculty to increase enrollment in existing nursing programs. When these programs reached capacity, the CNE was instrumental in securing Board support and funding to build a $2.5 million school of nursing for the California State University San Marcos (CSUSM) at the San Marcos Ambulatory Care Center site that is owned by PPH and leased to CSUSM for a nominal amount each year. The nursing school admitted 44 students in the fall of 2006 and is currently graduating more than 100 students per year.

With the supply side of the nursing shortage somewhat mitigated by these efforts, the CNE put forth a nursing recruitment strategic plan to the Board that called for the hiring and onboarding of more than 100 new graduate nurses in 2008 and 50 new graduate nurses in 2009 at the cost of $3.3 million. To support these new nurses, the PPH Center for Nursing Excellence (CNEx) created the New Graduate Nurse Residency Program. This program provides the new graduate nurses a year-long mentored experience to facilitate the transition from student to professional nurse. The New Graduate Nurse Residency Program was designed to assist the new graduate nurses to:

1. Demonstrate clinical competence at the advanced beginner level
2. Demonstrate effective decision-making skills and clinical judgment at the point of care
3. Incorporate research-based evidence into practice
4. Exhibit commitment to nursing through professional behavior
5. Develop an individual plan for ongoing professional development.

The New Graduate Nurse Residency Program is composed of 2 distinct phases:

Phase 1: during the first 12 to 16 weeks after hiring, nurse residents practice at the bedside under the supervision of an experienced preceptor. Included in this phase are 44 hours of classroom learning designed to assess and reinforce clinical skills and professional transition discussions to assist the novice in continuing their professional development.

Phase 2: for the remainder of the residency year, nurse residents receive a full clinical assignment but are provided an experienced "buddy" to serve as a resource and mentor. Continuous professional development support is provided through quarterly sessions that include the nurse resident, preceptors/mentors, and nursing education staff.

The CNEx also revised the preceptor training program and required all nurses interested in precepting new graduate nurses to attend these training sessions. This recruitment and retention strategy was highly successful, in that 92% of the new graduate nurses who were hired in 2008 are still employed by PPH after 18 months.

The onboarding and retention of these new graduate nurses as well as the significant reduction in turnover of all nurses, as noted in **Fig. 2**, allowed for the achievement of a subsequent nursing initiative that outlined a 10% over-hire strategy for all nursing departments. Hiring 10% more full-time equivalent employees than the allocated departmental budget allowed for coverage of unscheduled sick calls and extended leaves of absence without the use of costly premium pay shifts. Through these efforts the organization reduced its reliance on contract labor and overtime pay, resulting in a reduction in premium pay expenses by more than $5 million over 2 years.

Turnover for PPH RN vs. California Hospital Association – Southern California

Turnover	PPH RN	CHA RN SoCal	PPH All RN	CHA All RN SoCal
			Annualized Turnover	
Qtr 1 FY08	4.10%	3.40%	17.11%	12.90%
Qtr 2 FY08	2.53%	3.30%	14.40%	12.70%
Qtr 3 FY08	4.29%	2.70%	15.92%	12.60%
Qtr 4 FY08	2.71%	2.90%	13.63%	12.30%
Qtr 1 FY09	2.78%	3.30%	12.31%	12.20%
Qtr 2 FY09	3.52%	2.50%	13.30%	11.40%
Qtr 3 FY09	1.98%	2.20%	10.99%	10.90%
Qtr 4 FY09	2.19%	1.80%	10.47%	9.80%
Qtr 1 FY10	1.86%	2.40%	9.55%	8.90%
Qtr2 FY10	1.90%	2.00%	7.93%	8.40%
Qtr 3 FY10	2.40%	2.20%	8.35%	8.40%

* Excludes Per Diem Status
• Rolling 12 Months Reported Quarterly
• Includes Voluntary, Involuntary and Layoffs

Annualized Turnover Rates
PPH RN (Direct Patient Care) vs. CHA SoCal

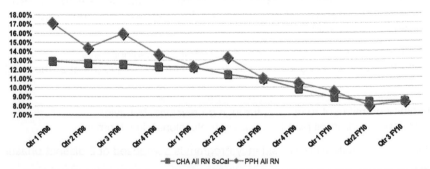

Fig. 2. Overall RN turnover for fiscal years 2008–2010. CHA, California Hospital Association; FY, fiscal year; Qtr, quarter; SoCal, Southern California.

COLLABORATIVE STRATEGIC PLANNING AND DECISION-MAKING STRUCTURE

PPH nursing maintains an integrated structure of interdisciplinary councils and committees to promote and improve system-wide quality of care through collaborative leadership and structural empowerment. The CNEx, an academic and service partnership developed to build nursing excellence capacity, provides mentorship and guidance to PPH nurses throughout the health system in the areas of quality, education, research, and informatics, in addition to facilitating and supporting the shared governance and decision-making structures and processes. Because the organizational infrastructure supports horizontal and vertical communications and decision making at the point of care, it is able to accommodate tactical changes quickly.

The collaborative leadership structure (**Fig. 3**) consists of a CLC that includes all nurse managers and above; advanced practice nurses; educators; the point-of-service staff nurse chair and cochair of the PPC; interdisciplinary partners from pharmacy, laboratory, imaging, dietary, and environmental services; and risk management and quality representatives. The PPC includes all point-of-service staff chairs from all of the Unit Practice Councils across the health system, the system CNE, director of the CNEx, clinical nurse specialists, and educators. The PPC meets for a general session once a month to address system-wide initiatives and is then divided into 5 working subgroups to address specific practice initiatives. These subgroups consist of evidence-based practice and research, practice, technology, patient and family education, and clinical consultants to the new building projects. The collaborative leadership structure and bylaws undergo annual review, evaluation, and revisions that reflect the continuing improvement and renewal of the structure and process.

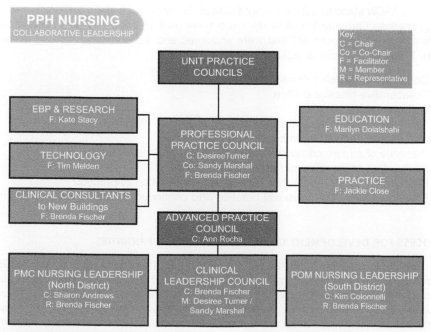

Fig. 3. Collaborative leadership structure.

EVIDENCE-INFORMED STRATEGIC PLANNING FRAMEWORK

The PPH nursing division's Magnet journey initiated in 2004 under the leadership of the CNE resulted in Magnet Recognition status for the health system in April 2009. Recognizing the Magnet designation as a milestone to nursing excellence, the CNE and the director of CNEx proactively embraced the new Magnet model in 2008 and incorporated its components into the strategic planning structure, process, and framework for the nursing division later that year. As noted in **Fig. 4**, this framework includes the nursing vision at the top of the document as a constant directional reminder. Underneath this vision are the health system's goals, objectives, and initiatives, organized by PPH's BSC domain, that nursing has a direct influence on achieving. Because the new Magnet model is solidly grounded in evidence, constantly striving for discovery and innovation, and flexible by design,[4] it was chosen to form the foundation of the strategic planning framework that would serve as a road map for nursing practice and research in the future. The Magnet components that comprise the left side of the framework include exemplary professional practice, structural empowerment, and transformational leadership. Knowledge, innovation, improvements, and empirical quality outcomes form the base of the framework.

Point-of-care staff nurse leaders at PPH had already embraced the American Association of Critical-Care Nurses (AACN) healthy work environment standards[5] and enthusiastically supported the inclusion of these standards into the strategic planning framework. These standards include:

1. True collaboration
2. Effective decision making
3. Appropriate staffing
4. Meaningful recognition
5. Authentic leadership.

These AACN standards form the right side of the framework along with the compatible American Organization of Nurse Executives (AONE) principles and elements of a healthy work environment[6] that were endorsed and supported by nursing leadership. The AONE principles include:

1. Communication-rich culture
2. Collaborative practice culture
3. Culture of accountability
4. Shared decision making at all levels
5. Presence of adequate numbers of qualified nurses
6. Presence of expert, competent, credible, and visible leadership
7. Recognition of the value of nurses' contribution
8. Recognition by nurses for their meaningful contribution to practice
9. Encouragement of professional practice and continued growth and development.

PROCESS FOR DEVELOPMENT OF NURSING STRATEGIC PRIORITIES

To identify nursing priorities for fiscal years 2009-2011 (beginning in July 2008), a participatory method guided by the components of the new Magnet model was used to support the nursing division's cultural transformation. A series of thoughtfully planned, sequential leadership development retreats for nurses at all levels were conducted in calendar year 2008 and they included tactical work on the nursing division's strategic plan. These retreats included the following:

1. The nursing executive team (NET) retreat, facilitated by the CNE, included the chief nursing officers from the 2 acute care campuses, the director of CNEx, the director of Home Care, the directors of the 2 skilled nursing facilities, and the chair and cochair of the PPC. This enriching retreat was a learning experience for both leaders and staff because the staff nurses gained an understanding of how high-level decisions were made, and the NET members gained a new insight on how their decisions affected the work of frontline nursing staff.
2. The PPC leadership development retreat, facilitated by the CNE and director of CNEx, included the staff nurses who served as chairs and cochairs of the Unit Practice Councils across the health system. The first half of the agenda covered topics such as developing leadership, advocacy, power and politics, communication, delegation, managing conflict, and quality (structure, process, and outcome). The last half of the agenda was devoted to tactical work on the nursing strategic plan.
3. The CLC leadership development retreat, facilitated by the CNE and the director of CNEx, included all nursing managers and above, advanced practice nurses, and educators, as well as interdisciplinary partners across the system. The first half of the agenda was organized around the quantum leadership work of Tim Porter-O'Grady, DM, EdD, APRN, FAAN,[7] with topics that included transformational leadership, designing high-performing clinical units, conflict management, complexity theory, and quality improvement and performance. The last half of the agenda was again devoted to tactical work on the nursing strategic plan.

Each of these retreats built on work from the previous retreat and allowed for input into the strategic plan from nurses across the health system while encouraging a deep understanding of the goals and priorities of the nursing division. Strategic planning and conversations included interdisciplinary partners, which resulted in newfound information and collaborative opportunities. This process created a new passion among the individuals and groups involved, which fueled their desire to grow professionally, share the successes, and exercise their pivotal role in shaping an exciting future. The goals and objectives associated with these 2008 retreats included:

1. Translating strategy into operational and tactical terms for ease of understanding
2. Aligning the nursing division with the overall strategies of the organization
3. Making strategy development the work of nursing at all levels of the organization
4. Mobilizing change through leadership at all levels in the organization
5. Making strategy a continuous renewal process.

The cascading assignments from these sequential retreats included team members developing tactics to carry out the strategies. These tactics outlined specific activities and functions that were intended to tie back the objectives of the organization. Because stakeholders were involved in every component of the strategy and tactic development process, they were fully invested in the process, which resulted in successful deployment and execution of the nursing strategic plan. Because the tactics were identified in an outcome format, the organization supported those behaviors, actions, and/or functions that facilitated achievement of the initiatives. In the past, there had been heavy emphasis on structure and processes but has more recently shifted to empirical outcomes. The cascade from strategies to tactics to performance creates an organized systematic mechanism that links important elements of the organization and creates a seamless connection to and between process and outcome.[7]

PPH Nursing Evidence-Informed Strategic Planning Framework FY09-11

PPH Nursing will be nationally recognized for setting the standard of nursing service excellence in practice, education, research, and leadership. Our Nurses are the Key.

Palomar Pomerado Health Balanced Scorecard Domains

	1. Financial Strength	2. Customer Service	3. Quality	4. Workforce Development and 5. Workplace Development
System Strategic Goals, Objectives & Initiatives Nursing has direct influence on achieving	Achieve *Aa bond rating* **1.1 Achieve profitability.** **Enhance clinical documentation** through completion of HealthworRx projects #5 (Clinical Documentation Program) and #28 (Present on Admission).	*Realize 90th percentile for physician and patient loyalty* **2.1 Develop loyal patients.** **Systematically implement best practices in patient loyalty.** **2.2 Develop loyal physicians.**	*Achieve national recognition for clinical quality and performance excellence including achievement of Magnet Designation and achieving the California Baldrige Award* **3.1 Demonstrate high quality, safe patient care. Systematically implement best practices to achieve reliable delivery of evidenced-based care.** **3.2 Optimize process efficiency and effectiveness. Systematically identify and improve key processes to increase reliable delivery of services.**	*Achieve national recognition as one of the top health systems in the country to work for, including achieving 90th percentile of employee engagement scores* **4.1 Attract, acquire and retain a high quality workforce. Implement a Workforce Strategic Plan.** **4.2 Create an environment of innovation, learning and professional commitment. Implement a systematic approach for management talent identification and succession planning for all managers and above.** **5.1 Provide the tools and equipment for optimal performance. Optimize Phase 1 Cerner system.**

"Roadmap for nursing practice and research into the future. Solidly grounded in evidence, flexible, and constantly striving for discovery and innovation."

	AACN Healthy Work Environment Standards	AONE Principles and Elements of a Healthy Work Environment
New Magnet Model Global Issues in Nursing & Healthcare Challenges Facing Nursing and Healthcare Today (with Forces)		
Exemplary Professional Practice	Skilled Communication	Communication-Rich Culture

Fig. 4. PPH nursing evidence-informed strategic planning framework.

	True Collaboration	Collaborative Practice Culture
4.1 Develop a recruitment and retention strategy that is linked to the organization's strategy. 4.1.1 Develop and implement a staff nurse clinical leader curriculum. 4.1.2 Develop and implement a consistent, participative practice of scheduling. 4.1.3 Develop an integrative program that provides a seamless transition for students at all levels to assume clinical roles. Owner: Sharon Andrews and Brenda Turner	Effective Decision-making	A Culture of Accountability, Shared Decision-Making at all Levels.
4.2 Develop and implement a comprehensive nursing communication strategy, to include Collaborative Leadership Bylaws revision, use of Intranet and Internet, and use of email. 4.2.1 Develop an interdisciplinary integration of the Collaborative Leadership Structure. Owner: Brenda Fischer	Appropriate Staffing	The Presence of Adequate Numbers of Qualified Nurses. The Presence of Expert, Competent, Credible, Visible Leadership.
5.1 Ensure Cerner Optimization Phase 1 implementation within the scope of the nursing division. Owner: Lorie Shoemaker	Meaningful Recognition	Recognition of the Value of Nursing's Contribution. Recognition by Nurses for Their Meaningful Contribution to Practice.
	Authentic Leadership	The Encouragement of Professional Practice & Continued Growth & Development

3.1 Ensure Present on Admission is contained in clinical documentation.
3.1.1 Develop education programs to ensure staff nurse competency to include Present on Admission and Hospital-Acquired Conditions.
Owner: Barbara Mayer and Opal Rainbold

3.2 Spread the use of Performance Improvement methodology to find solutions to practice and environmental issues.
Owner: Brenda Fischer

2.1 Develop a nursing customer service strategy, to include consistent scripting and use of whiteboards in each patient's room and activate consistent nurse leader rounding.
Owner: Kim Colonnelli and Sheila Brown

1.1 Ensure staff are informed on finances associated with staffing, supplies and other items that impact the nursing budget.
1.1.1 Ensure competency and shared accountability for achieving the financial targets of the organization and the department.
1.1.2 Activate consistent accountability for utilizing the Balanced Scorecard in management of the department and in communication to staff.
Owner: Lorie Shoemaker

Row categories:
5 Models of Care
8 Consultation and Resources
9 Autonomy
11 Nurses as Teachers
13 Interdisciplinary Relationships

Structural Empowerment
2 Organizational Structure
4 Personnel Policies & Programs
10 Community and the Health System
12 Image of Nursing
14 Professional Development

Transformational Leadership
1 Quality of Nursing Leadership
3 Management Style

Knowledge, Innovations, Improvements
Force 7: Quality Improvement
Empirical Quality Outcomes
Force 6: Quality of Care

Fig. 4. *(continued)*

In calendar year 2009, the retreats evolved into the first annual Nursing Summit, which included CLC and PPC, as well as staff from the quality division and organizational learning and development. The focus of the summit was on quality and patient safety, wherein functional groups from across the health system developed relevant work plans that were to be operationalized over the coming year. Data were provided to the Unit Practice Councils throughout the year on patient satisfaction, quality, and patient safety as well as to the Centers for Medicare and Medicaid Services core measures to inform decision making at the unit level.

The structure, process, and outcomes associated with the summit included building accountability into everyday unit level practice to emphasize high-performing clinical business units and create strategic plan awareness. The reporting mechanism for outcomes throughout the year included frequent monitoring of the initiatives via the online BSC tool, written documentation in the nursing annual report, and presentation by staff nurses at nursing practice council meetings and to the organization's BOD. Key to the successful outcomes was built-in flexibility, increased rigor and discipline around documentation and reporting, effective assimilation of information, and continual improvement of the process using the organization's plan-do-check-act performance improvement model.

CONTINUOUS RENEWAL OF THE STRATEGIC PLANNING PROCESS

The subsequent 2-year planning cycle for the nursing division's strategic initiatives began anew in 2010 after adoption of the organization's 4-year long-term goals, objectives, and initiatives. Sequential retreats are once again planned for the coming year as well as the second annual Nursing Summit. In the spirit of continuous renewal, this year's summit will include nursing students and leaders from the academic community to ensure alignment of curriculum with the long-term needs and goals of PPH as a whole and nursing in particular. This year's retreats and summit will map out the initiatives and tactics necessary to ensure successful transition into PPH's "hospital of the future" planned to open in 2012 as well as Magnet redesignation as a health system in 2013.

SUMMARY

This article described an evidence-informed strategic planning process and framework used by a Magnet-recognized public health system in California over a 5-year period involving nurses at all levels of the organization. This article includes (1) an overview of the organization and its strategic planning process, (2) the structure created within nursing for collaborative strategic planning and decision making, (3) the strategic planning framework developed based on the organization's BSC domains and the new Magnet model, and (4) the process undertaken to develop the nursing strategic priorities. Keys to the success of this organization's initiatives were the evolution of its collaborative leadership structure, the involvement and development of point-of-care staff nurse leaders, the alignment of its nursing division with that of the organization, and the continual renewal of its strategic planning process.

The more I read about self-renewing systems, the more I marvel at the images of freedom and the possibility they evoke. This is a domain of independence and interdependence, of processes that support forces we've placed in opposition–change and stability, continuity and newness, autonomy and control – and all in an environment that tests and teases and disturbs, and, ultimately, responds to changes it creates by changing itself.[8]

REFERENCES

1. Swayne L, Duncan W, Ginter P. Strategic management of health care organizations. 5th edition. Maine (ME): Blackwell Publishing; 2006. p. 3–44.
2. Koloroutis M. Relationship-based care: a model for transforming practice. Minneapolis (MN): Creative Health Care Management; 2004.
3. Kaplan R, Norton P. The strategy-focused organization: how balanced score card companies thrive in the new business environment. Boston: Harvard Business School Press; 2001.
4. American Nurses Credentialing Center. Application manual: Magnet Recognition Program. Silver Spring (MD): American Nurses Credentialing Center; 2008.
5. American Journal of Critical Care. AACN standards for establishing and sustaining healthy work environments: a journey to excellence; 2005. Available at: http://ajcc.aacnjournals.org/cgi/content/full/14/3/187. Accessed August 31, 2010.
6. American Organization of Nurse Executives. Healthy work environments: striving for excellence, volume II. 2003. Available at: http://www.aone.org/aone/docs/hwe_excellence_full.pdf. Accessed August 31, 2010.
7. Porter-O'Grady T. Interdisciplinary shared governance: integrating practice, transforming health care. 2nd edition. Sudbury (ON): Jones and Bartlett Publishers; 2009.
8. Wheatley M. Simple conversations to restore hope to the future. 2nd edition. San Francisco (CA): Berrett-Koehler Publishers; 2009.

The Implementation of the UHC/AACN New Graduate Nurse Residency Program in a Community Hospital

Karen L. Maxwell, MSN, RN-BC

KEYWORDS

- New graduate nurse • University health consortium
- Residency • Nursing internship • Internship and residency

Current nursing literature reports that the new graduate nurse turnover rate is 35% to 60% in the first year.[1–6] New graduate nurses now comprise approximately 10% of a typical hospital staff, and turnover is costly for hospitals.[7] According to the latest study by Jones,[8] examining the cost of nurse turnover adjusted for inflation, hospitals spend from $82,032 to $88,006 per nurse. These costs include pre-hire expenses of advertising/recruiting, closed bed/patient deferrals, temporary staff, overtime, productivity loss, hiring and post-hire costs of orientation/training, newly hired nurse's productivity, pre-turnover productivity, and termination.[8]

The National Council of State Boards of Nursing (NCSBN) conducted a survey in the fall of 2004 looking at the transition of the newly licensed nurse into practice. The study found that 20% to 50% of new graduates nurses did not feel they had been adequately prepared to provide direct care, administer medications, delegate tasks, supervise care by others, and communicate patient information to physicians.[9] The NCSBN 2004 survey found that residency programs play an important role in easing the transition of new nurses. This study concluded that there is a need to provide quality mentoring or orientation programs for new graduate nurses.[10]

St Joseph's Hospital of Atlanta, Georgia, a 410-bed tertiary acute care facility, has a reputation for innovation. St Joseph's has maintained Magnet designation for Excellence in Nursing Services from the American Nurses Credentialing Center (ANCC) since 1995, and takes great pride in the quality and caliber of the nurses within its

This work was sponsored by a grant from the William Randolph Hearst Foundation and the Keough Nursing Research Center at Saint Joseph's Hospital.
The author has nothing to disclose.
Saint Joseph's Hospital, 5665 Peachtree Dunwoody Road, Atlanta, GA 30342, USA
E-mail address: kmaxwell@sjha.org

Nurs Clin N Am 46 (2011) 27–33
doi:10.1016/j.cnur.2010.10.013
nursing.theclinics.com

organization. The Magnet Recognition Program was developed by ANCC to recognize health care organizations that provide nursing excellence and to support vehicles for investigating, testing, validating, and disseminating nursing practices and strategies targeted at improving either the environments for nurses or patient outcomes.[11] Although St Joseph's has met with considerable success as a nursing organization in areas such as shared governance, the new graduate nurse turnover rate was 50% or greater during the years 2001 to 2007. During that time, nursing leaders attempted to address this problem by enhancing the orientation of new graduate nurses through the implementation of the Dorothy del Bueno[12] PBDS Competency Assessment Program. As an additional intervention, in February 2006, a 10-week new graduate residency program was implemented. Unfortunately these changes did not result in the desired outcome of increased retention rates.

In October 2007, the nursing leaders at St Joseph's conducted a review of the literature and began a unique, internally developed model for new graduates as a 1-year internship program. Fifteen nurses were hired into the internship program as a cohort. These new graduates were not assigned to a particular unit in the hospital from the onset but were pooled together as a group. Each new graduate nurse rotated through 4 12-week assignments to different medical-surgical units in the hospital, with an option of transitioning to the Intensive Care Unit (ICU) or Emergency Department (ED) on the fourth rotation. The graduates also attended classes on 1 day a month, targeted toward particular content for further education and reinforcement of information. By the end of the first year 6 of the 15 new graduate nurses had resigned, resulting in a 40% turnover rate.

In March 2008, a clinical nurse specialist (CNS) was hired to manage a cohort of 29 new graduate nurses as a full-time role. The designation of this resource, and the recognition by the leaders of the organization regarding the impact of a CNS with population management and particularly with new graduate nurses, was a significant event. Charged with increasing the retention rate for new graduate nurses, the CNS developed class content and materials, organized rotations and preceptor classes, functioned as nurse manager for the cohort, and mentored and supported the graduates during their first year of employment. In August 2008, in response to ongoing cohort evaluations, the rotations for new graduates were decreased from the original 4 units to 3 units to provide more time for enhanced learning. Based on the new program, outcomes started to improve as 25 of the 29 new graduates hired in 2008 remained at the end of 1 year, resulting in a turnover rate of 14%. Continued analysis identified the lack of an evidence-based curriculum as a deficiency of the program.

THE UNIVERSITY HOSPITAL CONSORTIUM MODEL

In March 2009, St Joseph's Hospital joined the University Hospital Consortium (UHC)/ American Association of Colleges of Nursing (AACN) Nurse Residency Program, which provided an evidence-based curriculum and a database repository for comparison. The curriculum was developed by clinical and academic nursing partners from the UHC network as a research initiative. The UHC curriculum supports the essentials for practice as defined through the Magnet recognition program and many of the original 14 forces of magnetism.

The UHC/AACN Nurse Residency Program is based on Dreyfus' Model of Skill Acquisition and Benner's *From Novice to Expert in Clinical Nursing Practice*.[13] (Dreyfus S, Dreyfus H. A five-stage model of mental activities involved in directed skill acquisition. 1980, unpublished). Competencies expected to be demonstrated at the conclusion of the program include:

- Making the transition from advanced beginner to competent professional nurse in the clinical environment
- Developing effective decision-making skills related to clinical judgment and performance
- Providing clinical nursing leadership at the point of care
- Strengthening a commitment to nursing as a professional career choice
- Formulating an "Individual Development Plan" for the clinical role of the new graduate
- Linking research-based evidence to practice outcomes and then incorporating these principles into the care provided.[14]

Research had previously demonstrated that a 1-year residency model can be successful and that after 1 year, new nurses can develop the skills and knowledge needed to provide safe care if consistent processes, support, and content are in place.[15] At the end of 2009, 15,964 new graduate nurses had participated in the UHC/AACN Residency Program at a total of 56 sites, with 5 new sites joining in 2010. The overall retention rate for all participating sites as of 2010 is 95.6%.

The program incorporates a series of learning and work experiences to help the new graduate transition into their first professional role as a nurse, and is a multisite research study looking at the needs of the new graduate nurse. The curriculum is based on the *Essentials of Baccalaureate Education*.[16] In support of a desire for congruence with other participants related to educational standards, St Joseph's began to hire only baccalaureate (or higher) prepared new graduates into the residency program. Eighteen new graduate nurses were hired into the UHC/AACN Nurse Residency Program at St Joseph's Hospital in 2009, and 100% remained at the hospital at the end of 1 year.

UHC/AACN PROGRAM STRUCTURE

UHC uses a descriptive, comparative design and convenience sample of all new graduate residents hired to evaluate the program. Specific program characteristics for each participating site are reported among the facilities in the study to disseminate best practices as one of the benefits of participation. The program was originally developed as collaboration between an academic hospital setting and an affiliated school of nursing, and values partnership in all relationships as essential. Participating hospitals gain the added expertise of the university faculty, and the schools benefit from having access to the "lived" experience of new graduate nurses as they transition into practice. The partnership also helps validate that content from the *Essentials of Baccalaureate Education* has been met before graduation and that the residency program curriculum does not repeat the undergraduate content.[16]

The UHC/AACN program requires participating hospitals to have a partnering school or schools of nursing with dedicated faculty member involvement supporting the residency program. Each hospital is also required to establish an Advisory Committee to help maximize the success of the program. The advisory committee is made up of the chief nursing officer, school of nursing faculty, and representatives from managers, educators, preceptors, staff nurses, resident facilitators, and residents.[14] At a minimum, the academic partner should serve on the advisory committee, provide expertise to the residency coordinator on current academic curricula and anticipated changes, assess and determine appropriate instructional methodologies, help identify content experts, and serve as an educational resource. The primary role for the faculty representative is to support the hospital in developing and implementing the residency program. St Joseph's has relationships with many area schools of nursing. An advisory board was formed with participation of 4 local university schools along with the aforementioned suggested membership. The lack of one single academic partner has been identified as a weakness in the implementation of the UHC/AACN at St Joseph's. The schools involved in the initiative have regularly attended advisory committee meetings, but the complete implementation of the residency program has fallen to the hospital. Developing a stronger partnership with one academic institution would help to strengthen the residency program, and is a goal for the future.

The residency program is 1 year in length and is divided into 2 phases. Each phase is 6 months in duration. The content in both phases is framed around competencies including leadership, patient outcomes, professional role, critical thinking, and use of evidence-based practice. Based on the model, the curriculum may be customized to the organization, and is updated and revised on a 3-year cycle with the most recent revisions occurring in 2010.

A primary goal of the program is to improve the resident's critical thinking skills. To accomplish this, residents attend seminar days once a month for 6 to 8 hours. The seminar series begins with "Tales from the Bedside," which allows residents time to share concerns, fears, and frustrations, and to ask questions. Residents write a clinical narrative each month to share in class, and also write a reflection about their past month's experiences. Each activity contributes to the recognition and development of critical thinking in clinical situations.

PROGRAM EVALUATION

To evaluate outcomes of the residency program, all residents were asked to enroll as a participant in the UHC/AACN multisite research study; however, enrollment into the database was voluntary. Residents enter data directly through a password-protected portal on the UHC Web site. Approval was obtained from St Joseph's Hospital Institutional Review Board. Demographic data were collected on all residents and entered into the UHC database by the residency coordinator (the CNS). Residents were asked to complete The Casey Fink Graduate Nurse Experience Survey[2,17] on hire, at 6 months, and at 1 year. Participants are also asked to complete The Graduate Nurse Residency Program (GNRPE) evaluation[17] at the 1-year anniversary.

There are several potential limitations to the study. The sample is nonrandom and nonexperimental, and relies on self reports from an employee who may be considered vulnerable to participant response bias. The results of this study are generalizable to new graduate nurses employed in the inpatient academic hospital setting; however, further research would be needed to determine if there is applicability of the outcomes to new graduate nurses in other settings, including outside acute care hospitals.

DATA ANALYSIS AND OUTCOMES

The Casey Fink[2] Graduate Nurse Experience Survey comprises 4 sections including demographics, self-rating of skill competency, self-reporting confidence and comfort, and one open-ended question. The validity of the tool has been established by review of expert nurse directors and educators and has been shown to have a Cronbach alpha of .89. The survey measures 5 subscales: stress, perceived support, organizing and prioritizing, communication and leadership, and professional satisfaction.

Residents complete The Graduate Nurse Residency Program Evaluation (GNRPE) at the end of 1 year. The GNRPE comprises 3 sections and is designed to measure the overall satisfaction of residents with the program, how well program goals were met, and perceptions of support and subject topics.[17]

Demographic data and descriptive statistics along with statistical analysis are reported for each organization and in aggregate. Turnover rates have been measured at the end of the year and compared with the previous turnover rates of new graduate nurses at the other organizations. Narrative data have been collected and reported. Selected quotes have been included in this article.

Aggregate data are available to participating hospitals via the UHC Web site at all times. The results show the overall mean satisfaction score and the graduate nurse's self-reported satisfaction on a scale of 1 to 4 for the following 5 areas: support factor, organizing and prioritizing, stress, communication/leadership, and professional satisfaction. At the conclusion of the first year at St Joseph's, data analysis did demonstrate an increase from the beginning of the program to completion regarding the ability to organize and prioritize and in the areas of communication and leadership. The data for the stress scale showed a significant reduction between time of initial hiring and the 1-year scores in both groups. The level of support scores increased for the St Joseph's residents. Although the residents at St Josephs reported a reduction in professional satisfaction over this same period of time, this score remained relatively high, ranging from 3.4 to 3.52 on a 4.0 scale. This shift may be a result of the "reality shock" often experienced by new graduates during their first year in practice.[18]

The residents are asked to list the top 3 skills or procedures with which they are uncomfortable performing independently at each point of data collection. St Joseph's residents identified the following top 6 skills as the ones most uncomfortable when performing independently: code emergency response, vent care/management, chest tube care, central line care, blood draw/venipuncture, and tracheostomy care. These skills were addressed later in the program content and skills validation experiences.

Comments from June 2010 residents include:

Great opportunity.

I am thankful every day that I am in this Residency program. I am well aware that very few new grads get the experience that I am receiving in this program. I hope that our input in this study will allow more hospitals to create similar programs.

I am so glad that I was chosen and in return chose to do a residency program, it has been so helpful in so many ways. I wouldn't have my first year out of nursing school any other way.

The primary targeted outcome of the UHC program is new graduate retention. Other evaluative criteria include: (1) Do residents show significant improvement during the program in their confidence and competence, that is, support, organization, prioritizing, communication, leadership, and professional satisfaction? (2) What skills do the residents identify as the ones they are uncomfortable performing at the start and end of the program? As of August 2010, St Joseph's has had 18 nurses complete the UHC/AACN Residency Program. Nineteen nurses are currently enrolled in and are scheduled to complete the program in March 2011. St Joseph's has had 100% retention of the new graduate nurses hired into the UHC/AACN Nurse Residency Program from the first cohort.

SUMMARY

The UHC/AACN Nurse Residency Program is currently operational in 61 hospitals across the United States. St Joseph's Hospital has increased the new graduate retention rate to 100% in the first year since transition to the UHC/AACN Nurse Residency model from the reported 40% rate in 2007 prior to the initiation of the program. Residency programs do account for some additional cost to the traditional orientation programs usually offered to new graduates. However, Krugman and colleagues[18] found that the average budget for managing a program such as the National Post-Baccalaureate Graduate Nurse Residency Program is less than the costs required to advertise for and recruit two nurses.

The literature demonstrates that new graduate nurses do benefit from a specialized transition to practice program. Residency programs have led to higher recruitment and retention for this segment of the nursing workforce. For this reason it is important for institutions, and particularly nursing leaders, to understand the new graduate nurse experience so that they can develop effective strategies to ease transition.[1]

REFERENCES

1. Halfer D, Graf EI. Graduate nurse perception of the work experience. Nurs Econ 2006;23(3):150–5.
2. Casey K, Fink R, Krugman M, et al. The graduate nurse experience. J Nurs Adm 2004;34(6):303–11.
3. Pine R, Tart K. Return on investment: benefits and challenges of a nurse residency program. Nurs Econ 2007;21(15):13–8.
4. Beecroft PC, Kunzman L, Krozek C. RN internship: outcomes of a one-year pilot program. J Nurs Adm 2001;31(12):575–82.
5. Schoessler M, Waldo M. The first 18 months in practice: a developmental transition model for the newly graduated nurse. J Nurses Staff Dev 2006;22(2):47–52.
6. Poyton MR, Madden C, Roxanne B, et al. Nurse residency program implementation: The Utah experience. J Healthc Manag 2007;52(6):385–97.
7. Berkow JD, Virkstis S. Assessing new graduate nurse performance. J Nurs Adm 2008;38(11):468–74.
8. Jones CB. Revisiting nurse turnover costs: Adjusting for inflation. J Nurs Adm 2008;38(1):11–8.
9. Li S, Kenwood K. Report from the 2004 national survey on elements of nursing education. National Council of State Board of Nursing NCSBN Research Brief 2006;24. Available at: https://www.ncsbn.org/360.htm. Accessed October 19, 2010.
10. Kenward K, Zhong EH. Report of findings from the 2004 Practice and professional survey, Transition to practice: newly licensed registered nurse (RN) and licensed practical/vocational nurse (LPN/VN) activities. National Council of State Boards of Nursing NCSBN research brief 2006;22. Available at: https://www.ncsbn.org/360.htm. Accessed October 19, 2010.
11. American Nurses Credentialing Center. Recognizing nursing excellence application manual magnet recognition program. Silver (MD): American Nurse Credentialing Center; 2008.
12. del Bueno D. Performance management services incorporated. Available at: http://www.pmsi-pbds.com/. Accessed September 28, 2010.
13. Benner P. From novice to expert. Am J Nurs 1982;3:403–7.
14. University Health Consortium. Overview. In: Nurse residency program guide. Chicago: University Health Consortium; 2010.

15. Good CJ, Williams CA. Post-baccalaureate nurse residency program. J Nurs Adm 2004;34(2):71–7.
16. American Association of Colleges of Nursing. The essentials of Baccalaureate education. Washington, DC: American Association of Colleges of Nursing; 2008.
17. Krugman M, Bretschneider J, Horn P, et al. The national post-baccalaureate graduate nurse residency program: a model for excellence in transition to practice. J Nurses Staff Dev 2006;22(4):196–205.
18. Swihart D. The effective nurse preceptor handbook. Marblehead (MA): HCPro; 2007.

Professional Practice Model: Strategies for Translating Models into Practice

Jeanette Ives Erickson, RN, MS[a],
Marianne Ditomassi, RN, MSN, MBA[b],*

KEYWORDS

- Professional practice model • Magnet recognition
- Staff satisfaction • Professional practice environment

In the current health care climate, economic and cultural conditions have created an optimal opportunity to envision a new direction for nursing as a profession. Nurses, who have always led with standards undergirded by excellence, must now set the new description of what the nursing profession can be as well as identifying contributions to the care delivery model for the future. Toward that end, nurses find themselves in the formative stages of charting a new direction for the profession, regardless of the care setting. The articulation of a professional practice model provides a framework for setting this new direction and thus the achievement of exemplary clinical outcomes. In this article, the authors describe the evolution of the professional practice model at the Massachusetts General Hospital (MGH) and how the model continues to be evaluated and modified over time by the nurses within the system.

PROFESSIONAL PRACTICE MODEL

A professional practice model is a framework that allows nurses to clearly articulate contributions to practice from the profession. With a well-designed framework, nurses feel connected within the context of their relationships to the patient, to their own practice, to the roles of other providers in contributing to the plan, to other nurses, and to the institution. A framework and structure allows the nurse to better plan, manage, and adapt to change. A framework and the structures that ensue facilitate the identification of goals and strategies in addition to roles. Articulation of a model for the nursing

Disclosure: The authors have noting to disclose.
[a] Patient Care Services Operations, Massachusetts General Hospital, 55 Fruit Street, Bulfinch 230, Boston, MA 02114, USA
[b] Nursing and Patient Care Services, Massachusetts General Hospital, 55 Fruit Street, Bulfinch 230, Boston, MA 02114, USA
* Corresponding author.
E-mail address: mditomassi@partners.org

professionals within an organization provides a critical mass of energy to support resources, strength, and visibility within an often-complex structure.

The importance of a professional practice model has been recognized since the initial Magnet Hospital Study in 1983,[1] which articulated the salient elements of professional practice as autonomy, control over practice, and collaborative relationships with physicians. The MGH model builds on that foundation and incorporates findings from current research on organizational behavior, descriptive theory models, teamwork, and importance of a narrative culture. Each of these elements is a component of the practice of nursing at the MGH across care settings.

INITIAL PROFESSIONAL PRACTICE MODEL, 1996: VISION AND VALUES

In 1996, the initial model of professional practice at the MGH was framed by a well-articulated patient- and family-focused vision (**Fig. 1**). The unique contributions of each of the professional disciplines and support staff in collaboration with nursing brought special meaning to the relationships that were defined in the initial model, always keeping the patient at the forefront.

The vision acknowledging that the primary focus of the model was the patient, however, stressed the importance of preserving the integrity of the relationship between the patient and clinician as a key element for success. The vision clearly demonstrated the need for action in creating a practice environment that did not have insurmountable barriers, was built on a spirit of inquiry, and reflected a culturally competent workforce supportive of the family-focused values of the institution in practice outcomes.

Inspired by this vision, nursing leaders at the MGH launched new committees and initiatives in the late 1990s to publicly describe and exemplify the practice of nursing. This initiative helped to form an initial master plan for nursing focused on practice, organizational effectiveness, and collaborative decision making.

A clearly articulated set of values supported decision making and highlighted expressions in policies, practices, and norms of behavior. The development of a professional practice model enhanced and supported the values that leadership and staff followed and was a milestone for the initial journey to Magnet designation.

Components of a Professional Practice Model

Philosophy
A philosophy statement is derived from the values, principles, and beliefs, which support the individualized contributions of each discipline. Philosophy meant many

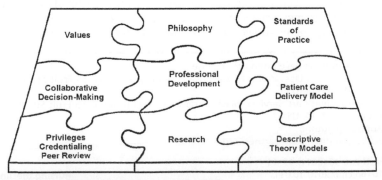

Fig. 1. The MGH professional practice model, 1996.

things within this particular model at the MGH. It was discipline specific and cited what each discipline believed in and what contributions the professionals wish to contribute to the whole. At the MGH, the philosophy of nursing focused on the patient care, education, research, and contributions of nurses to promote the quality and safety agenda.

Standards of practice

Standards are the practical application of values and philosophy. Standards of practice exist to ensure that the highest quality of care is maintained regardless of the professional providing the care or the experience level of those professionals. In a professional practice model, standards of practice support the "learner" or novice nurse as well as the experienced provider. For a provider lacking clinical mastery skills, standards of practice provide a structure on which to base and build practice and decision making. Standards serve as teaching tools by providing guidance in situations in which the provider may not be experienced. By serving as a teaching tool, standards of practice establish a level of expectation about care delivery and patient safety within an organization. Understanding the unique clinical needs of each patient and situation and appreciating the principles of critical thinking in applying standards is imperative to providing individualized, high-quality care. The ability to integrate clinical knowledge and standards of practice within a professional practice model is a competency common to experienced professionals.

Collaborative decision making

Collaborative governance is another component of a professional practice model. Collaborative governance is the decision-making process that places the authority, responsibility, and accountability for patient care with the practicing clinician. It is intended to empower professionals to control their own practice and create an opportunity to look at the contributions of each discipline and integrate them into the patient care delivery system. Collaborative governance should be a celebration of each discipline's contributions and is intended to support the staff in the elevation of practice to a more complex level. To ensure that collaborative governance is a success, the practice model framework should address a commitment of dedicated support. Examples of support include learning coaches for staff chairpersons, secretarial support for the teams, and resources within the literature.

Collaborative decision making is built on the premises of teamwork and team learning. The network of relationships between people who come together under a practice model structure can create strong bonds. Some of the most effective groups and teams at the MGH matured to a point where these groups and teams shared collaborative and interdependent relationships on multiple levels and within diverse practice settings. Members of these teams often described a sense of "feeling like we're making a difference."

Professional development

As the health care environment evolves and changes, professional development activities take on increasing importance in ensuring that nurses provide quality care as well as in providing a mechanism to attract and retain excellent clinicians. Professional development within a professional practice model supports the enhancement of leadership competencies as well as provides avenues for growth and career progression for nurses at all levels. Outcomes of professional development include mentoring, teaching, generating publications, conducting research and scholarly activities, as well as exemplifying patient care and family support. The context of professional development provides a framework for collaboration with nursing faculty colleagues in designing creative models for teaching, including a dedicated education unit where hospital nursing staff work with students and faculty to trial and monitor interventions supported by evidence-based practice and innovation.

Patient care delivery model

Design and definition of the care delivery model is one aspect of the professional practice model. The best care delivery model included in the optimal design promotes the highest quality while being cost-effective and patient centric. Nurses need to acknowledge that the health care world is changing but that their contributions will always be needed. The model for patient care delivery exemplifies the outcomes of the various components of the professional practice model because they are joined together in a way that can be described and replicated.

Privileging, credentialing, and peer-review

Another part of the professional practice model, privileging and credentialing processes, ensures that patients and their families receive quality care from competent nurses in all settings. The public trusts that there is a mechanism in place, which ensures that all nurses have the appropriate credentials. In addition to ensuring that the basics of licensure, certification, competency-based orientation, and training are in place, nurses should be encouraged to develop a professional portfolio. Nurses can use this portfolio when they represent their institutions externally or pursue advancement internally. Clinical narratives or exemplars are a key component of these portfolios at the MGH.

Peer review is an important component of privileging as well. This process supports autonomy and accountability for nursing practice within the organization. Through peer review, staff members have the opportunity as well as the responsibility to support each team member in improving both individual and organizational performance. An effective system of peer review and privileging within a professional practice model should ensure that the patient and their family members receive excellent care from competent providers.

Research

At the MGH, the practice model is based on knowledge, experience, tradition, intuition, and research. The implementation and support of evidence-based practice require a setting that promotes the acquisition and application of knowledge, provides access to new scientific knowledge, and fosters the ability of clinicians to use knowledge to affect patient outcomes.

Research is the bridge that translates academic knowledge and theory into clinical practice. Research dictates that evidence is a necessary prerequisite for the establishment of clinical practice, thus building the practice model. The goal of clinical researchers is to identify an issue of significant concern to the discipline of nursing and develop a substantial body of information related to that clinical phenomenon, which is scientifically vigorous and relevant.

Research-based practice within a practice model creates a spirit of inquiry that consistently challenges critical thinking of nurses at all levels. Translating the questions generated at the bedside into formal scientific hypotheses is a part of the continuum of professional development. Research must become an integral aspect of clinical practice as health care professions proceed from novice to expert. These research efforts define a systematic body of knowledge that guides professional clinical practice.

Theory-based practice

The challenges of the current practice environment present an opportunity to reflect on our practice, to articulate the "whys" of what we do. Understanding the philosophic, structural, and theoretical foundation of practice is an important component of professional development and the overall change processes that need to be taken to ensure that the practice environment is effective. As nurses develop into individual practitioners and collaborative colleagues, they find it exciting to share, explore, and challenge the theoretical perspectives used in the delivery of patient care.

REVISED PROFESSIONAL PRACTICE MODEL, 2006

Ten years after the articulation and implementation of our initial professional practice model at the MGH, nurse leaders critically reviewed the model of professional practice and identified that updates were indicated to meet the current demands of health care delivery (**Fig. 2**). Updates to the professional practice model framework are described in the following sections.

Narrative Culture

The creation of a narrative culture has been transformational at the MGH. Over time, clinical narratives have become part of the fabric of professional life in the organization. Narratives are part of the application process for the clinical advancement program, awards, and annual performance review.

Clinical narratives have been introduced as an effective vehicle to share and reflect on clinical practice. Benner[2] cites that, "narrative accounts of practice reveal the clinical reasoning and knowledge that comes from experiential learning. Clinical narratives have been reported to help the practitioner in understanding their practice, including strengths and impediments, and to see and share the clinical knowledge of peers."

Although putting pen to paper allows clinicians to see their practice in a different light, it is also a springboard for dialogue with colleagues and clinical experts. Through the very important process of dialogue, and thus communication, clinicians are asking questions that prompt them to delve deeper into their thinking and motivation.

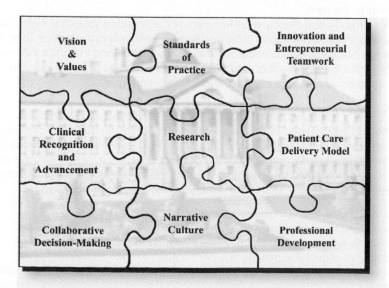

Fig. 2. The MGH professional practice model, 2006.

Clinicians might ask themselves the following questions. What were my concerns about his patient in this situation? How was this situation similar to situations I have experienced in the past? How was it different? What did I learn? These questions allow clinicians to enter into the clinical situation from a different perspective, see it in a different way, and, perhaps, identify different interventions and strategies.

Clinical narratives can be difficult to read when they do not describe what is considered to be "perfect practice." At the MGH, it has been found that those are the narratives one needs to write and talk about because they describe the realities of care and the environment in which care is being provided. The practice model has evolved to be open to all stories and the dialogue that follows, thus creating and sustaining the highest quality of care.

Clinical Recognition and Advancement

Clinical recognition and advancement have been found to be effective retention tools within our organization. The Clinical Recognition Program at MGH developed as clinicians reviewed narratives written by clinicians and identified themes and criteria, which applied to the 6 disciplines, including nursing, physical therapy, occupational therapy, respiratory care, speech-language pathology, and social work. Themes including the clinician-patient relationship, effective patterns of clinical decision making, teamwork, and collaboration emerged. In narratives, clinicians spoke of advocacy and clinical risk taking and on how these constructs influenced clinical practice at the MGH. Analysis of these themes helped establish a set of professional behaviors and attributes that act as developmental milestones, which have now been implemented as a component of the professional practice model.

The theoretical foundation of the Clinical Recognition Program is the Dreyfus Model of Skill Acquisition. Developed by Dreyfus and Dreyfus,[3] this model described how, in the acquisition and development of a particular skill, individuals pass through the 5 stages, novice, advanced beginner, competent, proficient, and expert. The word "stage" is crucial as it relates to the recognition program at the MGH because it reinforces the idea that clinicians must master each stage or level or development before progressing to the next.

Central to the Clinical Recognition Program is the reflective process, which allows individuals to incorporate theory with practice, shaping clinical practice over time. This process helps individuals understand their experience and integrate information in a meaningful way. Reflective practitioners committed to lifelong learning have enabled us to advance and sustain excellence in patient care.

Innovation and Entrepreneurial Teamwork

Innovation and entrepreneurial teamwork are critical to the creation of a professional practice environment that embraces change. As nurses and health care clinicians, we need to innovate and make certain that the delivery of patient care and structures that support it change to meet the changing populations we serve. Several key assumptions guide the work at the MGH with regard to innovation:

- Our employees are our biggest assets.
- Innovation takes great leaders.
- Imagination is necessary and fun for innovation to occur.
- Collaborative decision making is a core value.
- A professional practice environment is the foundation on which we will build our future.
- Patient-centered care is the key.

Together, questions about beliefs, values, and traditions and how these will affect innovation, are addressed. These clinicians must also address the designing of the ideal environment for innovation, the changes that need to occur for the success in regard to this ideal environment, and the best way to capture insights from practitioners at the bedside.

Patient Centeredness

Patient centeredness is the most critical piece of the revised professional practice model and is strategically placed in the center, touching all other components. The ability to efficiently and effectively care for patients and families requires the support of an array of resources, programs, and processes. At the MGH, the professional practice model now embraces the 6 pillars of quality and safety described by the Institute of Medicine[4]:

- *Safety*: We will work to ensure no needless death, injury, or suffering of patients and staff.
- *Effectiveness*: Our care will be based on the best science, informed by patient values and preferences.
- *Patient-centeredness*: All care will honor the individual patient and the respective patients' choices, culture, social context, and specific needs.
- *Timeliness*: We will waste no one's time and will create systems to eliminate unnecessary waiting.
- *Efficiency*: We will remove all unnecessary processes or steps in a process and streamline all activities.
- *Equity*: Our work will ensure equal access to all.

EVALUATING OUR PROFESSIONAL PRACTICE MODEL

Evaluation of the professional practice model Is truly integrated into our practice environment; we use 2 methodologies, internal and external. Internally, we have administered our Staff Perceptions of the Professional Practice Environment Survey to nurses and clinicians across patient care services every 12 to 18 months since 1997. This tool

- Provides an assessment of 8 organizational characteristics (**Table 1**) determined to be important to clinician satisfaction
- Allows clinicians the opportunity to participate in setting the strategic direction for patient care services
- Trends key information
- Provides feedback on strategic goals
- Identifies frequency, preparation, and access to resources in managing common patient problems
- Identifies opportunities to improve the environments for clinical practice (**Table 2**).

This psychometrically sound tool has been implemented locally, nationally, and internationally.[11,12]

Externally, MGH applied for Magnet recognition to validate that we have a strong professional practice model. Magnet recognition by the American Nurses Credentialing Center is the highest honor awarded to health care institutions for excellence in nursing services. Grounded in research, this intensive review is the ultimate confirmation that a supportive professional practice model and environment is thriving within an organization.

Table 1
Patient care services, organizational characteristics, and definitions

Organizational Characteristic	Definition	Source
Autonomy	The quality or state of being self-governing and exercising professional judgment in a timely fashion	Aiken et al[5]
Clinician-MD relations	Relations with physicians that facilitate exchange of important clinical information	Aiken et al[5]
Control over practice	Sufficient intraorganizational status to influence others and to deploy resources when necessary for good patient care	Aiken et al[6]
Communication	The degree to which patient care information is related promptly to the people who need to be informed through open channels of communication	Shortell et al[7]
Teamwork/Leadership	A conscious activity aimed at achieving unity of effort in the pursuit of shared objectives	Zimmerman, Shortell, Rousseau, Duffy, Gillies, Knaus, et al[8]
Conflict Management/ Handling disagreements	The degree to which managing conflict is addressed using a problem-solving approach	Zimmerman et al[8]
Internal work motivation	Self-generated motivation completely independent of external factors such as pay, supervision, and coworkers	Hackman and Oldham[9]
Cultural sensitivity	A set of attitudes, practices, and/or policies that respects and accepts cultural differences	The Cross Cultural Health Care Program[10]

The updated Magnet recognition model[13] is composed of 5 elements, transformational leadership; structured empowerment; exemplary professional practice; new knowledge, innovations, and improvement; and empirical outcomes. The heightened focus on demonstrating the outcomes and effects of nurses' work challenges leaders within a Magnet organization to critically review and improve the structure and processes that support care delivery.

For Magnet-recognized organizations or for organizations on the journey to Magnet recognition, the Staff Perceptions of the Professional Practice Environment Scale may be an effective tool to measure baseline and ongoing perceptions of clinicians' impressions of their professional practice model, which is aligned with the 5 model elements of Magnet recognition. Administration of the survey over time provides a greater understanding of opportunities to enhance clinical practice because outcomes are trended. At the MGH, this information has provided direction about

Table 2
Patient care services survey: issues and strategies

Staff Perceptions Survey Issue (Survey Year)	Interventions/Outcomes
Need for recognition of clinical work (1998)	The chief nurse charged the Professional Development Committee within Collaborative Governance with the responsibility to design an interdisciplinary clinical recognition program. The first-of-its-kind interdisciplinary clinical recognition program was implemented in 2002
Requests for additional educational opportunities (1998)	The Center for Clinical and Professional Development was expanded to include orientation, training, and continuing education opportunities for clinical and support staff
Concerns identified with supplies and linen (2000)	Established Materials Management/Nursing Task Force
Need for more in-services on various cultures to deliver culturally competent care (2001)	The Culturally-Competent Care Lecture Series was launched to augment the daylong culturally competent care curriculum offered. Developed unit/department culturally competence care resource manuals
Request for increased Nursing Director availability (2001)	Nursing Director span of control was analyzed and reduced where appropriate
Need to enhance communication (2002)	Numerous communication strategies used; increased use of email to improve communication; created the "Fielding the issues" column in departmental newsletter, Caring Headlines, to present timely information in a question and answer format
Concerns identified regarding support from the Department of Food and Nutrition (2002–2003)	Food and Nutrition/Nursing Task Force established.
Request for assistance with regard to public speaking and talking to the media (2004)	Launched media and public speaking programs through The Center for Clinical and Professional Development.
Request for conflict resolution skills training (2005–2006)	Developed workshops to present information/skills to work with a multigenerational workforce, negotiation, and preparing for, and actively engaging in, difficult conversations.
Need to identify strategies to support the aging nursing workforce (2006)	Conducted multisite qualitative study designed to explore concerns of the aging nursing workforce. Hosted Coming of Age Summit on November 15, 2007, a think tank regarding issues facing the aging nursing workforce
Need to align work of collaborative governance committee with emerging strategic issues (2008)	Redesigned collaborative governance communication and decision-making committee structure to align with strategic goals
Need to develop tools to facilitate the ability of nurse leaders to correlate key data, eg, nurse sensitive indicators, patient and staff satisfaction data (2010)	Developed a relational crosswalk of core measures to provide at-a-glance information about unit- or department-based metrics

the support structures that are necessary to hardwire the 6 aims of the Institute of Medicine into practice.

At the MGH, the way we think about, organize, and deliver care is evolving as health care delivery and nursing practice are evolving. Nurses are the most important discipline in connecting all the pieces of the new care delivery model. At the MGH, we feel that a refined professional practice model is one construct that enables our staff to continue the integration and continued growth of theory as an essential element of practice. For any professional practice model to be effective, nursing leaders must understand, embrace, and master the skills involved in setting up the structure and then leading others through resources and support to achieve the desired state of practice. This practice is a journey nurses and other members of the health care team must take together to chart the future of health care and care delivery.

REFERENCES

1. McClure ML, Poulin MA, Sovie MD, et al. Magnet hospitals: attraction and retention of professional nurses. Washington, DC: American Nurses Publishing; 1983.
2. Benner P. From novice to expert: excellence and power in clinical nursing practice. Menlo Park (CA): Addison Wesley; 1984.
3. Dreyfus HL, Dreyfus SE. Five steps from novice to expert. In: Mind over machine. New York: Free Press; 1986. p. 16–51.
4. Institute of Medicine. Crossing the quality chasm: a new health system for the 21st century. Washington, DC: NationalAcademy Press; 2001.
5. Aiken L, Sochalski J, Lake E. Studying outcomes of organizational change in health services. Med Care 1997;35(Suppl 11):NS6–18.
6. Aiken L, Havens D, Sloane D. (2000). The Magnet Nursing Services Recognition Program: a comparison of two groups of magnet hospitals. Am J Nurs 2000; 100(3):26–36.
7. Shortell S, Rousseau D, Gillies R, et al. (1991). Organizational assessment in intensive care units (ICUs): construct development, reliability and validity of the ICU nurse-physician questionnaire. Med Care 1991;29:709–23.
8. Zimmerman J, Shortell S, Rousseau D, et al. (1993). Improving intensive care: observations based on organizational case studies in nine intensive care units. Crit Care Med 1993;21(20):1443–551.
9. Hackman J, Oldman G. Motivation through the design of work: test of a theory. Organ Behav Hum Perform 1976;16(2):250–79.
10. The Cross Cultural Health Program. Introduction to cultural competence. Available at: http://www.xculture.org. Accessed September 22, 2010.
11. Ives Erickson J, Duffy M, Gibbons P, et al. Development and psychometric evaluation of the professional practice environment (PPE) scale. J Nurs Scholarsh 2004;36(3):279–84.
12. Ives Erickson J, Duffy ME, Ditomassi M, et al. Psychometric evaluation of the revised professional practice environment (RPPE) scale. J Nurs Adm 2009; 39(5):236–43.
13. American Nurses Credentialing Center. Announcing a new model for ANCC's magnet recognition program, 2008. Available at: http://cms.nursecredentialing. org/Magnet/NewMagnetModel.aspx. Accessed September 22, 2010.

Transforming Organizational Culture Through Nursing Shared Governance

Karen Profitt Newman, EdD, MSN, RN, NEA-BC

KEYWORDS

• Shared governance • Nursing autonomy • Decision making

There is a widely used expression in leadership circles that suggests, "Culture trumps strategy every time." Baptist Hospital East (BHE), a 519-bed acute care community hospital in Louisville, Kentucky, has a long history and reputation for excellence in nursing and as a consultant once stated, "A culture of nice."

The vice president and chief nursing officer (CNO) came into the organization in 1999, with a strong belief in a transformational leadership style and empowerment. Although the organizational structure of BHE had historically been a traditional hierarchical model, the nursing division had been decentralized for many years. It became quickly apparent that decision making regarding nursing practice was primarily a top-down process driven by the senior nursing leadership group called the Nurse Council. The Nurse Council was chaired by the CNO and comprised of directors from across the organization. This council encompassed leaders from the behavioral health, oncological, neuroscientific, and cardiovascular service lines; surgical services; emergency, critical care, maternal child, medical-surgical, and rehabilitation services, as well as the directors of risk management, education and professional practice, clinical informatics, quality and outcomes management, and home health, all of whom are nurses. In the spring of 2000, the CNO conducted a doctoral dissertation research study in the organization, examining nurses' perceptions of leadership styles and the relationship between leadership styles and empowerment. The findings of the study indicated that nursing leaders in the organization predominantly used a transformational leadership style; staff members had a strong sense of empowerment but thought that nursing leaders should be more innovative and exert a greater upward

Disclosures: The author has nothing to disclose.
Department of Administration, Baptist Hospital East, 4000 Kresge Way, Louisville, KY 40207, USA
E-mail address: knewman@bhsi.com

Nurs Clin N Am 46 (2011) 45–58
doi:10.1016/j.cnur.2010.10.002
0029-6465/11/$ – see front matter © 2011 Elsevier Inc. All rights reserved.

influence in the organization. The data suggested that nurses recognized and valued transformational nursing leaders who are innovative, influential, and empowering.[1]

Despite these findings, as well as a high level of nursing satisfaction, the culture was such that staff expected decisions to be made at the management level and was reluctant to participate in projects or initiatives beyond direct patient care. Nurses freely verbalized their opinions but did not demonstrate consistent commitment to participate in problem solving or process improvements. The culture was not unlike that of many organizations in which the nurses' locus of control had become so narrow that they preferred to do only the most functional and routine activities and had become content with the status quo of predictable and ritualistic functional activities of nursing.

The CNO and nursing leaders recognized that engaging and empowering nurses, the hallmark of SG, has been associated with good management for many years. They had a vision for professional nursing practice in the organization and understood that a retooling of leadership capacity and skill was required to successfully implement SG and sustain it as a way of life. Nursing leadership set the context for engaging staff as well as managers in that vision and provided support for this priority of a more participative form of governance. Although the CNO and nursing leaders were inspired to transform the culture, they understood that the commitment to a new form of shared decision making would need to be valued by and arise from the staff rather than be a top-down goal.

In his definitive book on SG first published in 1984, Tim Porter O'Grady articulated a different mental model for relationship and leadership. Nursing shared governance (NSG) provides a framework for the professionalization of nursing, provides a broader distribution of decision making across the profession, and allocates decisions based on accountability and role expectations.[2] Shared governance (SG) defines staff-based decisions, accountability, roles, and ownership of staff in those activities that directly affect nurses' lives and practice.[3] Although NSG is a somewhat ambiguous concept with a vast application, examining it from the perspective of structure, process, and outcomes can more clearly outline a successful strategy for implementation and growth.

EVOLUTION OF A VISION FOR SG
Identifying the Need for SG

Assessing staff interest in NSG began months before the organization took its first steps toward formalizing a structure. The American Nurses Credentialing Center's Magnet Recognition Program was introduced to staff and leadership, discussing the principles of the program in short conversations across a variety of venues. Simultaneously, nurse leaders were gauging interest and readiness to begin developing the structure that would be required in a Magnet culture.

The first employee engagement survey was facilitated by an external vendor in November 2003. Although survey results indicated that nurses were more engaged and satisfied than the hospital's employee base overall, registered nurses (RNs) responded with lower values in key priority items such as:

- "My ideas and opinions count"
- "The organization values my contribution"
- "In this organization there is open and honest two-way communication"[4]

The survey results validated nursing leadership's perception that the nursing division was ready for real change in the professional practice culture. Survey results showed an overall nursing engagement index (EI) of 76%, indicating that 76% of respondents agreed with the following 3 questions: (1) overall, I am extremely satisfied with this organization as a place to work, (2) I would gladly refer a good friend or family member to this organization for employment, and (3) I rarely think about looking for a new job with another company. The EI measures the overall level of employee engagement with the employer. The top 3 areas in which opportunities existed as identified by the 79% of nurses participating in the survey were increased opportunity to provide input in decision making, improved communication overall, and a clearer more progressive vision for the future of the nursing division.

In late 2003, the CNO engaged The Prine Group, a consulting firm regarded for their work on NSG implementation and Magnet readiness and preparation. They met with small focus groups of nurses at all levels of the organization to assess interest and readiness to pursue Magnet designation and to perform an informal strengths, weaknesses, opportunities, and threats (SWOT) analysis of the nursing practice environment. The consultants noted themes regarding lack of communication and input into decision making, and nurses articulated the desire for a greater role in decision making on issues that would affect their professional practice. The Essentials of Magnetism[5] were evaluated by focus groups noting that "concern for the patient is paramount" was strongly evident in the organization.

The CNO had established the practice of hosting nursing town hall meetings. These open forums were conducted shortly after the 2003 employee engagement survey and focus groups and further confirmed the desire of nursing staff to have a voice in practice discussions. Because of these various feedback venues, nursing leadership had a clear and compelling message from staff that they desired a process for shared decision making regarding their practice. Staff also communicated strong support for taking formal steps toward Magnet designation. About 91% of nurses attending town hall meetings favored embarking on the journey to Magnet designation.

Ensuring Commitment

Town hall meetings with the CNO had validated the results of the employee engagement survey and focus groups and were used as the catalysts to encourage staff in sharing the vision and commitment to participate in decision making. Armed with substantial data indicating overwhelming staff support for a change in the nursing practice environment, nursing leadership began to engage key advocates. Administrative buy-in was the foundation to the long-term success of a legitimate NSG structure. It was critical that the organization's executive team endorse the financial investment needed to implement and sustain NSG. This endorsement required education on SG for the nursing staff as well as nurse managers, budgeted dollars for meeting and project time, and the projected expense of implementing potential changes that would result from the work of SG. Of equal importance, executive leadership needed to understand and embrace a change in mind-set, which would support staff involvement in decisions. No less important was understanding by the medical staff as to what NSG was and the value this framework would bring to patient care.

Senior nursing leadership embraced the feedback regarding the need for a participative style and initiated educational programs to increase the knowledge and understanding on SG. Arguably the most pivotal players in the success of NSG are nurse managers. Recognizing their importance, proactively engaging their support was essential. Nurse managers and senior nurse leaders were provided education on SG theory and concepts including various models, the role of leadership, and the benefits and challenges of implementing NSG. In-depth education regarding change theory was also provided. This same group completed a SWOT analysis of the existing nursing culture and practice environment, similar to the work of the focus groups. Managers completed an environmental assessment of their individual units focusing on clinical competence and skills, learning environment, culture and systems, and staff talent. With the assistance of the Prine Group, analysis of the environmental assessment was completed for each unit. As a result, each manager began developing a framework for both organizational NSG and unit-based SG (UBSG). The factors included:

- What features to include in an SG structure
- Who would be involved in developing the structure and model for SG
- What would be the first priority or focus for SG
- How would UBSG integrate with the overall SG process for the nursing division
- What would the time line be for implementing the SG plan.

These combined efforts laid the foundation for a structured plan for NSG implementation with a clear awareness of the existing gaps and potential barriers. Through focus groups, survey results, town hall meeting takeaways, and educational sessions with nursing leaders, the consultants provided a comprehensive report and recommendations:

1. Educate/increase awareness of Magnet concepts, commitments, and cultural transformation required
2. Move nursing division toward an SG decision-making structure
3. Develop strategic and tactical plans for enhancement of the nursing professional practice environment in accordance with the Magnet Recognition Program standards.

Engaging Champions

Great leadership was witnessed in staff nurses as many continued to provide input regarding this change (NSG) to their practice environment. It was essential to garner staff support that would be needed to implement and guide a change of this magnitude. Setting this transformation as nursing leaders' highest priority sent the message to staff that they were valued and trusted to have a greater role in decision making regarding their practice.

The NSG Steering Committee was formed to guide the development and implementation of a NSG model. The membership included the CNO, selected senior nurse leaders, advanced practice nurses, educators, and staff nurses from all clinical areas. Members were peer selected based on the following criteria: (1) role model for excellence in leadership; (2) respect of peers; (3) optimistic and progressive mind-set; (4) ability to represent area and area goals and integrate with overall hospital goals; (5) ability to communicate, seek input, educate, and update; (6) demonstration of personal responsibility and accountability; and (7) ability to partner with others to achieve shared goals. Concurrent with the development of the NSG Steering Committee was the formation of the Magnet leader group to begin guiding the Magnet journey in areas outside NSG.

A critical partner to support the implementation of NSG was the human resources (HR) department leadership. Invitation was extended to the vice president of HR department to serve in an ad hoc advisory capacity to the NSG Steering Committee. Collaboration with the HR department was vital because boundaries related to wages, benefits, conditions of employment, hours, and workplace environment were delineated. Understanding that NSG was consistent with the organization's investment in human capital, the HR department was an essential partner in this endeavor as well as the Magnet journey. The NSG Steering Committee served until its purpose and function were subsumed into the council structure.

DEFINING A STRUCTURE FOR SG
Examining Best Practices

The NSG Steering Committee reviewed existing models and best practices with a goal of developing a model that was congruent with the existing culture. The NSG Steering Committee completed an extensive review of the literature on SG, attended seminars on SG, and engaged in discussion with organizations having a mature NSG. The group frequently revisited the goal of NSG—to support the relationship between a nurse and patient by increasing the role of the nurse in decision making. Consideration was given to the appropriate scope of authority and the need to drive accountability.

After several months of research and discussion, the NSG Steering Committee selected the councilor model. Initially, this model involved the creation of 3 separate function-based councils, namely, Quality and Research, Practice, Education and Professional Development, reporting to both an oversight council, which is the Coordinating Council, and a Senior Nursing Leadership Council. This approach was consistent with the organizational culture and mission. This new structure also provided for the absorption of several well-established nursing-based committees such as Policy and Procedure, Nurse Manager/House Manager, and Nursing Quality.

The NSG Steering Committee formally chartered the councils and outlined membership needs. Best practices were studied, and much dialogue ensued regarding the most effective composition and size for a council. Most areas and units in which nursing is practiced were asked to designate 1 representative per council for the 3 function-based councils. Select small units (eg, Radiology triage, Pediatrics) were combined with other similar service units for representation, reducing potential strain on staffing for council meetings and activities. Each council also included nursing leader liaisons as well as advanced practice nurses. Membership complement resulted in each function-based council having approximately 35 members. The Coordinating Council was designed to include the elected chair and cochair from each of the 3 function-based councils, as well as a limited number of nursing leaders; membership was voluntary. NSG was formally introduced to the organization through a kickoff event and an educational seminar for council members in May 2004.

Outlining Roles, Scope, and Limitations

The next step for the NSG Steering Committee was the creation of NSG bylaws to guide council activities and scope of influence. Sample bylaws from other organizations were reviewed and they provided a context and reference point for the development of the organization's bylaws. Initial bylaws provided for membership composition and a schedule for reappointment or replacement of members, attendance parameters, and scope of authority for the council. In addition, the bylaws outlined the membership and decision-making processes. Finally, to ensure that all eligible and interested staff were provided with an opportunity to participate in the councils, the membership would be rotated. As each council met for the first time, a chair and cochair were chosen via consensus and a meeting schedule was identified. Each council also developed its purpose statement and list of priorities.

Garnering Nursing Input

As with any change, support for the new idea comes best through demonstrating the benefits. NSG brought small and great outcomes that in turn generated increasing nursing support for this previously foreign concept. For example, in the first year of NSG, the nursing councils:

- Drafted and approved their adjunct mission, vision, and values to guide professional practice
- Adopted a professional model of care and nursing theoretic framework
- Revised and expanded the nursing clinical ladder program
- Assisted with the implementation of bar-coded medication administration technology.

Over time, nursing staff easily integrated into a new professional practice model defined by shared decision making. This integration also meant that nurses often forgot how they practiced before the implementation of NSG, sometimes failing to recognize and appreciate the great transformation that had occurred in their practice environment.

Each time an issue or opportunity was unearthed, conscious effort was made to ask, "Where should we route this?" or "What council needs to look at this?" Senior nursing leadership had become highly cognizant of the importance of and need for staff-level input. Most inspiring was observing how the conscious effort to include staff in decision making gradually became enculturated - SG had become part of the organizational DNA.

ESTABLISHING THE PROCESS FOR SG INFLUENCE
Education and Communication

Within the first year of initiation of NSG, several educational offerings were provided to the council cochairs as well as members. Educational needs were identified including how to plan and conduct meetings, consensus building, taking minutes, and facilitating change. The organization was fortunate to possess the internal resources to provide professional development in these areas. Early efforts also focused on enriching the knowledge of general SG theory and principles through regional conference and National Magnet Conferences. Annual education for SG chairs and UBSG chairs continues.

One of the greatest challenges for successfully sustaining and growing NSG is communicating the goals and results. With a staff of more than 1200 nurses, communication became and remains a focal point and a challenge. Communication venues also provide the opportunity for ongoing education on NSG. In summer 2005, the Education and Professional Development Council proposed the reincarnation of a nursing newsletter that had been suspended years earlier. The "Stethoscoop" became a primary means for communicating anything regarding nursing but especially the work of SG. Stethoscoop was and continues to be staff written and produced. The publication, much like the NSG structure, has undergone change and maturation. The original black and white photocopied 2- to 4-page newsletter has evolved into a 26- to 30-page glossy full-color news magazine published quarterly. Stethoscoop chronicles the work of each NSG council and showcases the accomplishments of 2 or 3 UBSG councils in each issue.

Communication is an area that councils constantly look for improvement and new ideas. The Coordinating Council developed an issue submission form whereby staff electronically submit a concern, problem, or idea that they would like SG to consider. The Coordinating Council reviews submissions and directs them to the appropriate council for review. In addition, the councils implemented a "takeaway" form. Council chairs create a 1-page takeaway form at each meeting and share it electronically with the members. The takeaway form articulates the key work in progress of the council, any council projects underway, and recent council achievements.

Most recently, each council created an internal Web page. The council Web page includes meeting schedules, member contact information, council specific documents, and completed takeaway forms. The Web pages link to each other as well as to the Magnet Web page, allowing easy access to the end user to current information on any council.

With NSG in place for more than 6 years, the Education and Professional Development council felt the need to archive the council's work. The council created a council time line outlining the work of the council and its achievements since the council was created. The time line was presented to the Coordinating Council that adopted it as a council best practice. As a result, each council created their own time line. These time lines are updated annually and they provide a historical account at a glance of the great works of NSG.

Fostering Autonomous Decision Making at the Organization and Unit Levels

In concert with the implementation and evolution of an enterprise-wide NSG framework for decentralized decision making, work began on fostering the same process at the individual unit level. A diverse group of staff nurses and nurse managers had the opportunity to attend a conference on SG with Tim Porter-O'Grady. This conference was a fundamental step in expanding and solidifying the SG structure. The knowledge gained was used to initiate new ideas and processes for successful unit-based decision making. Insights were shared with other nurse managers, the SG councils, and the UBSG leaders during the initial UBSG training.

Individual units began their work on establishing UBSG councils whose purpose is to proactively address unit-level issues to improve patient care, safety, and quality. Focus is on practice enhancement and strategies for improvement. Unit representatives from the Quality, Education, and Practice councils disseminate information to the UBSG chair or cochair to ensure that house-wide efforts are shared with nurses across the organization. In addition to developing processes, practices, and policy and procedures that are unit specific in nature (eg, scheduling policy), unit-based councils are responsible for developing improvement strategies addressing key nursing initiatives such as patient satisfaction and core measures outcomes. Using this organized approach ensures that key nursing strategic initiatives are addressed at the unit level, with participation and ownership of the key individuals influencing their success (the direct care nurses and caregivers themselves). Each UBSG council is structured and operated according to the design of the unit staff, allowing the council to serve the unique needs of each unit and better fit the individual unit culture. Membership composition is defined by the unit as well. Members include nurses as well as nursing support and ancillary staff. The UBSG framework recognizes that many issues can be solved and improved at the unit level through the inclusion of all team members and stakeholders.

NSG implementation does not occur without obstacles and challenges. One of the most difficult challenges encountered was fostering autonomous decision making within the boundaries and scope of SG. Staff were accustomed to a top-down decision-making structure and had to learn how to participate in decision making. The learning curve was significant for some staff. Simply sharing recommendations was not a practice staff was accustomed to. As the point-of-care providers, they were best suited to give input that could make a meaningful difference in the quality of care provided and/or the practice environment. Developing an understanding of the difference between consensus and majority rule was also necessary. Nurses also had to nurture their spirit of inquiry, that is, asking questions such as why a process was designed the way it was, how to deliver better care or more efficient service, and what strategies could enhance nursing practice in the organization. Some of the best outcomes of NSG have been a result of questioning practice norms and challenging the status quo. As staff witnessed changes, they grew increasingly more inclined and adept at inquiry and innovation.

Providing Tools and Resources for Success

Availability and accessibility of resources was important in facilitating the work of the councils. In partnership with the information technology and HR departments, Internet access was expanded to SG council members to facilitate research, literature reviews, and exploration of best practices. Clerical support was identified for assistance in preparation of meeting agendas, minutes, and documents. The organization's medical librarian was introduced to the SG structure and integrated throughout council activities. The librarian provided vital education to council members on search engines, data repositories, and tools available to simplify their efforts toward evidence-based practice. The CNO engaged 2 regarded, doctorally prepared, academic-based nurse researchers to serve as consultants to the nursing division in the areas of nursing research and evidence-based practice. These experts have assisted in elevating research, provided education, and aided in developing a research mentor group. Education in the areas of research and evidence-based practice was prerequisite to productive work from any of the councils, particularly the Quality and Research and Practice councils.

Lessons Learned

The lessons learned from the implementation and growth of NSG are vast and ongoing. SG is dynamic, with the framework evolving continuously as an organization grows, needs change, ideas emerge, and lessons are learned.

Structural changes

The NSG structure has remained intact but changes have been made along the journey. Early in the original SG model, the Coordinating Council consisted of all nurse managers and directors. This design quickly yielded some concerns. Because there was no forum for council chairs to convene, there was duplication of effort among the councils. There were occasions when the inexperienced councils would bring forward a recommendation, without a well–thought-out plan for implementation or consideration of potential unintended consequences. Hence, council members and chairs sometimes thought that their time and effort was in vain. A forum of more manageable size was needed for the chairpersons to discuss issues from the councils and gain feedback for resolution.

Nursing leadership determined that to truly empower the councils and prevent frustration and rework, the Coordinating Council needed restructuring. The new Coordinating Council consists of council chairs for Education, Practice, and Quality/Research, a nurse manager, and a director and serves as a clearinghouse for individual council assignments and activities. With this change, the lines of communication have improved. All council chairs are aware of what is happening in other councils, and managers better understand their role in facilitating decision making at the councilor level. This revised structure and process is demonstrative of the continued evolution of transformational leadership within the nursing department. The nurse leaders and CNO supported a change to improve the functioning of the SG structure.

Another significant structural change occurred after the organization's Magnet site visit in late 2008. Appraisers suggested that consideration be given to separating the

Quality and Research Council into 2, fostering the ability of each group to have a unique identity and focus. This change was enacted in early 2009 with strong support from the Quality and Research and Coordinating Councils (**Fig. 1**). Therefore, the Research Council has facilitated greater focus on generating bedside science, promoting nursing research endeavors, and broadening understanding of nursing research across the enterprise. Establishing a separate Research Council has also further helped differentiate research from evidenced-based practice. Although research and evidenced-based practice are closely linked, additional education regarding the differences between them was needed. The Quality Council has become more involved in monitoring and reporting metrics and in collaborating with the Practice Council to improve outcomes related to nurse-sensitive indicators. The link between the work of the Quality Council and the Research Council remains important, and ongoing attention to communication between the 2 councils is essential to avoid fragmented efforts. Most recently, the Coordinating Council membership was expanded to include additional staff representation from each council.

Initial efforts to ensure representation of each council from every nursing area proved challenging for some units. As a result, some units attempted shared membership, appointing 2 nurses from a unit to rotate attendance and responsibility on a given council. Although this approach was effective for a few select units, it was generally not a strategy that worked for the council or the unit. The "buddy system" for council representation requires a high level of commitment and exceptional communication on the part of the sharing members. Without these elements in place, units can be isolated from the work of councils and progress on initiatives can -languish.

BHE continues to work toward strengthening the UBSG councils. As such, the lessons learned continue to emerge. However, one decision that has proved to be positive was the creation of centralized function-based organizational councils, followed by the incremental development of UBSG councils. This approach provided opportunity to learn from the implementation of a limited number of groups, with consistent support from leadership before moving to the more diverse, abundant, independently formed and managed UBSG councils.

Boundaries and roles

Boundaries and roles are the 2 areas in which many lessons have surfaced. Boundaries define the scope and limits of NSG. Although these are clearly articulated in the SG bylaws, there have been occasions of ambiguity around a specific issue. By way of example, the Education and Professional Development Council spearheaded an initiative to improve the preceptor program focusing on outcomes of enhanced retention, satisfaction, and quality of care. Through review of the literature and research of best practices, it was evident that some organizations provided monetary incentives to preceptors. The council drafted a formal proposal outlining numerous strategies for improving the preceptor system, including reward and recognition of preceptors. Line item in the proposal was a suggestion that preceptors be additionally compensated for the hours they spend precepting. As this recommendation was in the realm of wages and benefits, it extended beyond the boundaries of SG. Reeducation was provided to council members regarding the scope of SG influence. The HR department collaborated with the council and the proposal was resubmitted, suggesting that compensation for precepting be incorporated into the annual salary analysis conducted for the organization by an external vendor. This suggestion was accepted and included in the next salary survey of regional pay practices. This example underlines the importance of a leadership liaison to guide each council when boundary issues become apparent.

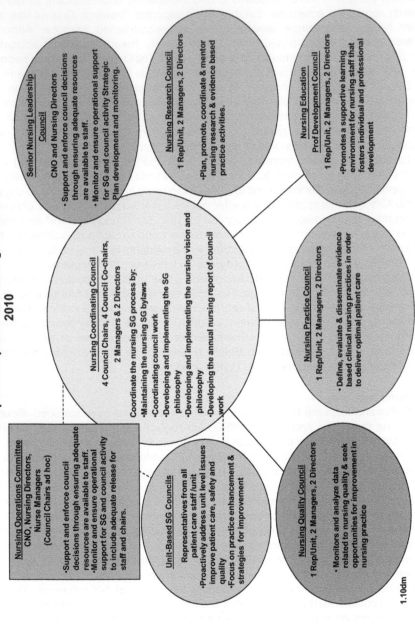

Fig. 1. BHE SG model 2010.

Another challenge has been clarifying the role of management in SG, particularly at the unit level. Some nurse managers have struggled with understanding their role in the SG structure; therefore, ongoing communication and education regarding the role of management in SG is necessary. The Coordinating Council assigned each of its members to serve as mentor to designated UBSG councils. Mentors have received additional education in SG and assist in resolving SG issues at the unit level and in increasing the work of the UBSG council to focus on meaningful outcomes.

Outcome rigor

A final area of focus has been steadily raising the bar on the issues and projects that councils, both centralized and unit based, work toward. Councils have been encouraged to address goals aimed at enhancing patient outcomes. Initially, many UBSG councils were focused on social efforts to build morale (eg, birthday parties, staff night out, pet bulletin boards). Although important to team building, these endeavors did not fulfill a significant aspect of SG. It was important, however, not to quash enthusiasm and to build confidence at the unit level. As UBSG councils realized what they could achieve on small issues and were recognized for their work, they were energized and engaged to take on more substantive issues. Three years ago, UBSG councils began presenting formal reports to the Nursing Operations Group. This group consists of all nurse leaders and members of the Coordinating Council. When these presentations began, it was common to hear reports of holiday parties and efforts toward cleaner waiting rooms. As groups matured in their focus, the reports began centering on topics such as strategies to improve patient satisfaction scores, initiatives to increase the number of certified nurses in the unit, and efforts to enhance collaboration with support departments. The transformation represents the maturation of UBSG structure.

ACHIEVING OUTCOMES FROM SG: EXEMPLARS OF EXCELLENCE

As Porter-O'Grady so well stated: "Staff-driven decision-making is a strong indicator of excellence. The outputs of this shared framework are innovation and creativity that leads to excellent patient care."[6] BHE has greatly benefited from the adoption and maturation of NSG. Some achievements have been small in scope but significant in effect, whereas others have been comprehensive projects with house-wide implications. Outcomes have been generated at the unit and organizational levels. The following is a small sample of the many exemplars of excellence resulting from NSG.

Patient Outcomes

Falls reduction

The Joint Commission National Patient Safety Goal No. 9 addresses the need to reduce the risk of (patient) harm resulting from falls.[7] In the autumn of 2008, injury caused by falls became a Centers for Medicare and Medicaid Services (CMS) "never event." Organizational outcomes data indicated that the Neuroscience Unit (5 Park Tower) consistently reported the highest rate of falls in the organization. The 5 Park UBSG council requested to serve as the pilot unit for the falls team's evidence-based rounding initiative. The 5 Park UBSG developed and piloted a rounding log, making needed changes as requested by staff. Substantial effort was invested in unit education on rounding. The 5 Park unit demonstrated a significant reduction in unit falls (**Fig. 2**). Parallel increases in patient satisfaction scores were achieved. These remarkable results were formally shared with nursing leadership and throughout the NSG councils. The rounding process, inclusive of the comprehensive education, was adopted house wide. The 5 Park UBSG has since taken the rounding initiative a step further,

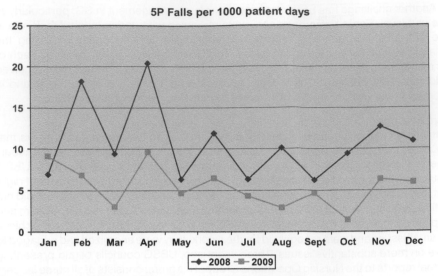

Fig. 2. The 5 Park falls per 1000 patient-days 2008 versus 2009.

introducing shift change walking rounds to improve handoff communication between caregivers.

Improving congestive heart failure patient education
Improving heart failure outcomes continues to be a challenge for acute care and home health care providers. A task force was formed led by representatives from UBSG on the Progressive Care Unit to examine opportunities for enhancing congestive heart failure (CHF) care and improving patient education, with the intent of reducing readmission. Based on review of the literature, the group agreed that the present evidence-based education was a logical first step in addressing the challenges.

The group developed a comprehensive CHF education booklet, initiated a study to compare the knowledge level of patients with CHF before and after implementation of the tool, improved the process for nutritional and home health consults for patients with CHF, and modified processes to enhance accuracy of information at discharge regarding medication compliance. Subsequent to the work of this group, the organization has demonstrated an improvement in the CMS core measure score for CHF discharge instructions from 71% (in 2009) to 83% (data to date in third quarter 2010).

Nurse Outcomes

National Database for Nursing Quality Indicators satisfaction
BHE has participated in the National Database for Nursing Quality Indicators (NDNQI) RN Satisfaction Survey since 2007. Participation rates have been consistently high and steadily increased (2007, 58%; 2008, 67%; 2009, 79%; 2010, 80%). Responses on the 2010 survey indicated scores higher than the NDNQI mean of 34 out of 42 indicators, improving from 2009 in 40 variables. The primary focus area is the practice environment scale (PES). The PES used in the survey is endorsed by National Quality Forum, an accepted authority that develops and implements national strategies for health care quality measurement and reporting. Practice environment is a term that encompasses all the elements of the work environment that contribute to or impede the practice of professional nursing. On a 4-point scale, the PES score for BHE nurses

Table 1
Baptist Hospital East NDNQI survey response rate and PES results

Calendar Year Data	2007 BHE Results	2008 BHE Results	2009 BHE Results	2010 BHE Results	2010 NDNQI Mean All Hospitals
Survey Response Rate/Number of RNs responding	58% (577)	67% (588)	79% (824)	80% (879)	84%
PES					
Mean PES Score	2.90	2.94	3.05	3.09	2.95

has consistently increased (**Table 1**), exceeding the mean for all hospitals surveyed each year.

Safe lifts and handling
The nurse wellness subgroup was created as a subgroup of the Practice Council to promote and enhance the physical, psychosocial, and spiritual well-being of the BHE nursing staff. One issue the subgroup addressed was the rising rate of musculo-skeletal injuries (MSIs) associated with patient lifts and transfers. The American Nurses Association white paper on Safe Patient Handling and Movement served as a guide to the group's work. After reviewing the best practices and lifting products available, the group piloted minimal lift equipment on 3 different units. Equipment purchase recommendations were presented to executive leadership in the fall of 2008 and approved. Policy revisions and education were completed over the next 8 months. From 2008 to 2009, a 25% reduction in MSIs was demonstrated in the inpatient units, with one large medical-surgical unit reporting no MSIs for the entire year. For the first half of 2010, inpatient units have reported 36 MSIs for an annualized rate of 72, a 34% reduction. The overall cost of MSIs has decreased by $250,000 from 2008 to 2009.

Organizational Outcomes

Engagement scores
The organization conducts employee engagement surveys approximately every 18 months. Scores for the nursing division before the implementation of SG revealed an EI of 76% (in 2003). The EI reflects overall long-term commitment to the organization. A year after establishing an NSG structure, the EI for nursing was 84%, representing a statistically significant 8% increase.

Nurse retention
Since the implementation of NSG, the organization has enjoyed modest but favorable reductions in RN turnover. Before NSG, the RN turnover remained stagnant at 13% to 14% annually. Most recent fiscal year to date data indicate an organizational RN turnover rate of 10%.

SUMMARY

The work of SG is not easy and cannot be accomplished overnight. It requires organizational commitment of time, resources, and staff accountability. It is critical to be strategic in the implementation of NSG. The importance of patience with the process cannot be overstated. Skepticism is to be expected and can be motivational. Successful implementation requires a well–thought-out plan, a time line, and inspired leadership. The accomplishments and outcomes of SG should be celebrated and heralded.

The past 6 years have demonstrated significant growth and maturation of SG at BHE. It has been an evolutionary process at the broad organizational level as well as at the individual unit/department level. The framework of SG has engendered nurse autonomy; staff are increasingly more confident in decision making and view themselves as empowered decision makers. They have come to view the SG structure as a primary means for providing feedback and affecting practice changes. Through SG the nursing culture has been transformed, once again "trumping strategy."

The nurses at this organization are not only permitted but expected to practice autonomously consistent with professional standards. Nurses here are confident in their clinical knowledge and stalwart advocates for quality patient care. Nurses willingly engage in confronting issues and challenges in care delivery and in identifying and bringing forth issues and ideas including through their structure of a strong and active share governance model that empowers nurses to recommend changes to policy and practice. The number and variety of issues that nurses and nursing staff have influence is impressive. Staff projects a "can do" attitude and is self-directed in their unrelenting passion and pursuit of excellence.[8]

ACKNOWLEDGMENTS

My sincere thanks to Darla Meredith, RN, MSN, Director of Education and Professional Development at Baptist Hospital East for her leadership and support throughout the development and implementation of shared governance at our organization and the preparation of this article.

REFERENCES

1. Newman K. The impact of leadership style & empowerment on organizational structure [dissertation]. Spalding University, Louisville (KY); 2001.
2. Porter O'Grady T, Finnigan S. Shared governance for nursing: a creative approach to professional accountability. Gaithersburg (MD): Aspen Publishers, Inc; 1984.
3. Swihart D. Shared governance: a practical approach to reshaping professional nursing practice. Marblehead (MA): HCPro, Inc; 2006.
4. Kenexa Human Capital Management Corporation. Proceedings of a proprietary survey. Baptist Hospital East employee engagement survey, 2003.
5. Kramer M, Schmalenberg C. Development and evaluation of essentials of magnetism tool. J Nurs Adm 2004;34(7):365–78.
6. Porter O'Grady T, Hawkins M, Parker M. Whole-systems shared governance: architecture for integration. Gaithersburg (MD): Aspen Publishers, Inc; 1997.
7. The Joint Commission. Comprehensive accreditation manual. Oakbrook Terrace (IL): Joint Commission Resources, Inc; 2010.
8. American Nurses Credentialing Center. Magnet recognition program: Magnet appraisers summary report to Baptist Hospital East. Silver Spring (MD): American Nurses Credentialing Center; 2008.

Empowering Nurses Through an Innovative Scheduling Model

Pamela A. Maxson-Cooper, MS, BSN, RN, NEA-BC

KEYWORDS

- Innovative registered nurse scheduling model • 7/70
- Nurse satisfaction • Nurse retention

All professionals expect their career working schedule to be consistent and predictable. However, predictability and control over the hours nurses choose to work within the acute care hospital are not usually possible. Routinely, schedules are developed by staffing schedulers, lead nurses, or computer-generated programs that are posted up to 3 months in advance. Holidays or personal requests for days off must be submitted within a designated timeline, and senior nurses within the units usually get priority. Yet, more control over work–life balance choices is what the professional seeks, especially those employees from generations "X" and "Y," which is no different among the nursing workforce.[1] As a matter of fact, probably even more important and challenging, is that nurses must cover patient needs 24-hours per day, 7 days per week in acute care. This leaves nurses feeling dissatisfied with their schedules, and retention may become a challenge for employers. Peter Buerhaus, PhD, RN, FAAN,[2] Director of the Center for Interdisciplinary Health Workforce Studies in the Institute for Medicine and Public Health at Vanderbilt University Medical Center, reports that many factors influence the decision of a nurse to leave nursing, and inflexible scheduling is one of the major reasons cited.

As national averages of registered nurse vacancy rates increased from 12% to 22% from 2002 to 2007, turnover rates decreased from 29% to 17%. Due to this trend and other issues, the focus for employers has turned toward retention of experienced nurses as a strategic priority.[3] In part due to the recent economic downturn, there appears to be a brief respite from these trends, as registered nurses remain working or return to the workforce to preserve benefits or supplement income. Buerhaus and colleagues[2] predict that, as the economy recovers, nurses who recently returned to the workforce or who worked additional hours to supplement their income will leave the workforce again. Those who delayed retirement will start considering and

The author has nothing to disclose.
Froedtert Health, 400 Woodland Prime, Suite 311, N74 W12501 Leatherwood Court, Menomonee Falls, WI 53051, USA
E-mail address: pmaxson@froedterthealth.org

executing their exit strategies from the workforce once their retirement income is replaced or more secure.[4]

Recent studies regarding the cost of nurse turnover have reported that it ranges from $22,000 to $64,000, while yet other sources estimates the cost at 1.3 times the salary of the departing nurse.[5] Costs include advertising, recruitment, replacement of the vacancy, orientation, and decreased productivity. Resources used in replacing nurses from avoidable turnover could better be applied toward educational reimbursement, rewards and recognition, and clinical advancement programs, thus supporting retention strategies. The benefits of retention have been identified to include patient safety, quality of care, patient satisfaction, nurse satisfaction, and nurse safety. Ensuring safe staffing levels and offering flexible work schedules, along with job sharing and good wages, are all strategies that have been identified as nurse satisfiers and factors in registered nurse retention.[5] Focusing on retention, thus controlling cost of recruitment and necessary replacements through an innovative, scheduling pattern based on staff empowerment has been a key strategy at Froedtert Hospital in Milwaukee. This article describes the setting, the history, the response, the success of this unique scheduling program, and the story of one nurse leader within this Magnet designated setting.

HISTORY

When Froedtert Hospital opened its doors in 1980, the organization offered a unique and innovative scheduling model to both full-time and part-time staff RNs. Known as 7/70, the program of 10-hour days, 7 days on and 7 days off has been the primary core scheduling pattern for Froedtert registered nurses for the past 30 years. This extremely popular plan has contributed significantly to increasing retention levels and decreasing turnover costs. One of the unexpected outcomes of this unique pattern has been a consistent supply of experienced nurse applicants as word spread in the community, which translates to registered nurse candidates waiting for open positions in many areas. The program has been recognized as an important factor in the quality and continuity of patient care at Froedtert Hospital.

Froedtert Hospital began as a tertiary hospital, opening its doors within the Milwaukee community where several hospitals already had been established. The new director of nursing (DON) was immediately challenged to recruit enough registered nurses to care for approximately 200 patients a day. The DON introduced this unique scheduling pattern to the nursing community and within 3 months had recruited the first group of qualified candidates. As one of the first nurses in this new program, I recall how extremely excited I was to be able to work this unique schedule, manage my responsibilities as a single parent, and complete studies for my bachelors of science in nursing while being able to work full-time. The hospital is affiliated with the Medical College of Wisconsin, which affords the benefits of an academic environment to the employees including accessible classroom resources. The predictability of the schedule allowed me to attend class every other weekend and still work full-time, with every other week off to study, attend class, and have time with my daughter. The predictability also provided maximal flexibility by allowing me to plan my school and personal schedules up to a year ahead of time and count on those times on or off shift.

Most hospitals require nursing staff to work every other weekend, or the organization may hire added staff to cover the shifts at a premium. This additional cost is often prohibitive in a tight economic environment. In addition, added system cost may be realized through decreasing interruptions in patient continuity and diminishing the negative impact to patient safety often attributed to multiple handoffs.[6] As the model was implemented later and compared by patients with that of other hospitals in the community, the patients were often surprised yet pleased that the same registered nurse cared for them on each shift throughout their stay at Froedtert Hospital. This realization served to build a sense of trust and confidence in the continuity of care among the patient population. Personally, the scheduling model allowed me to prioritize time with my growing daughter and plan events and activities with her, thus supporting a deep bond between us as she grew.

Upon completion of my degree, I was promoted to the DON role, where I was able to hire and manage the staff to work the same scheduling model I had participated in as a staff nurse. The role of the DON was transitioned to a vice president/chief nursing officer role, I was promoted, and I began to lead the hospital's journey to Magnet designation which became a reality in 2006. The innovative scheduling program was key evidence in Froedtert's demonstration of staff empowerment, shared governance, and professional growth opportunities for the nursing staff.

As Froedtert Hospital has become nationally recognized throughout the Magnet community, I have networked with other leaders who are interested in evaluating and implementing the 7/70 model. From my experience, applying the schedule to existing staff can often have a negative impact on personal and professional schedules. The smoothest implementations have been those where staff are hired into new departments or positions and start the 7/70 model from the onset.

HOW DOES IT WORK?

The 7/70 system is based on three overlapping 10-hour shifts during 7 consecutive days. During the overlap of time, two shifts of nurses manage admissions, discharges, and transfers; care for very complex patients; attend meetings; and receive any necessary education. Day and evening shifts are 10.5 hours in length due to a 30-minute unpaid meal break. However, night shift works 10 hours of paid time including meal break in recognition of the fact that there are fewer places to access during night shift for an entire hour break off the unit. The staffing model provides 30 hours of registered nurses in a 24-hour day, hence 6 hours of overlap during shifts.

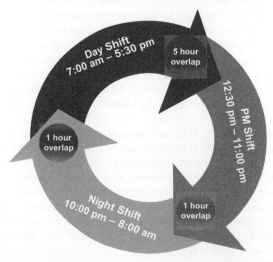

This scheduling permits overlap of all shifts, with the largest bulk of time during the afternoons. Nurses work 70 hours in a 2-week pay period versus the more frequently reported 80-hour pay periods in other facilities. Alignment of the overlapping shifts during the busy periods assists in maximizing staffing resources at Froedtert Hospital.

Also, nonlicensed clinical support staff members work these schedules, which has resulted in two cohesive teams divided into an A team week and a B team week. The team model is supported in the rotation and scheduling patterns, because 1 week the members of A team work, while during the same week the entire B team is off for 7 days. From the date of hire, registered nurses can count on 26 weeks off a year, along with the ability to accrue 1 to 3 weeks vacation annually depending on longevity. Three holidays fall within each team's rotation, so the six holidays are always covered, as are the weekends with staff on regular time and not premium pay. Registered nurses are hired into set hours and do not rotate shifts. The stability of this scheduling model has added to registered nurse satisfaction, and the formation of the team of caregivers has resulted in better satisfaction and continuity for the patients.

Night shift registered nurses report satisfaction with the work schedule, because they can be awake and home with their families for 7 days straight. Also, they can plan for the nights they will not be home far in advance to arrange for child care services. The nurses appreciate the time for respite and recreation.

Nurses are provided the flexibility to have days of work switched if the trade does not result in overtime. During holidays, leaders within the organization tend to be even more accommodating with regard to trades and possible overtime. Since registered nurses are paid for 70 hours instead of 80 as scheduled full-time (SFT) staff, they are able to return to work for one extra shift on their off week to help cover sick and vacation time at regular salary. This scenario results in 10 hours of straight time as compared to depending on overtime for relief coverage, which has resulted in an organizational savings. There is no mandatory overtime at Froedtert Hospital.

As this scheduling pattern was created it became apparent about one-third of every unit's RN staff are interested in picking up an extra shift and often look for these opportunities to expand their paychecks. Scheduled part-time staff (SPT) can job share one full-time position, therefore splitting the 7-day work schedule. Typically, one registered nurse works 3 days, while the other 4 days, and the rotation is reversed during the second week. Therefore they each work 70 hours in 4 weeks.

The overlap time is primarily used to plan care for complex patients, shared governance activities, to plan or participate in educational offerings, and to attend department meetings. Meals breaks are covered by the same amount of staff for the shift, so there is no delay in patient needs or care. Assignments are done as a team as they begin their shifts, and there is always a primary and secondary registered nurse for each patient during afternoon overlap. This team approach ensures there is always a professional nurse present for each patient and decreases hand-off concerns.

Surveys of registered nurse staff satisfaction are completed annually by a contracted national vendor; however, work schedules have not been found to be directly correlated to the general question responses. To assure the primary 7/70 work schedule is a satisfier for registered nurses at Froedtert Hospital, the nursing staff members are asked to complete a brief focused internally developed survey every 3 to 4 years. The most recent survey results yielded a 53% response rate (n = 364), with adequate participation noted from all shifts and departments (**Box 1**). The responses validated the satisfaction of the nursing staff with this type of scheduling pattern; comments are listed in **Box 2**.

Box 1
Highlights of the 7/70 registered nurse survey

67.3% chose to work at Froedtert Hospital because of the 7/70 schedule.
82.96% continue to work at Froedtert Hospital because of the 7/70 schedule.
90.38% like working 7/70.
71.98% believe the overlap of shifts helps provide high-quality care.
92.86% felt the continuity of known scheduled days, same patients, helps them provide high-quality care.
70.33% felt they had more opportunities to advance their professional growth.
60.44% believe overlap helps them to attend meetings and participate in shared governance.

REGISTERED NURSE VACANCY AND TURNOVER

Froedtert Hospital has grown from the original days and now employs over 1600 registered nurses. From 2004 through 2009 the vacancy rate decreased from 4.25% to 2.07%. In comparison, the 2009 average statewide registered nurse vacancy rate was 9.1%.[5] In further analysis, no significant patterns have been apparent in any one department related to vacancy or turnover. Nursing turnover increased slightly, rising from 7% to 11%; however, this was also a period of significant change within the organization related to the Magnet journey. Expectations and accountabilities, along with the implementation of shared governance, were all systems changes with impact on the nursing staff. The turnover rate at Froedtert Hospital does, however, routinely fall well below reported national averages for registered nurse turnover.

COSTS

Each full-time registered nurse works 70 hours in 2 weeks or .875 FTE (full time equivalent) with full-time benefits. This scheduling pattern does not increase the overall FTE requirements but applies the total FTEs in a specific scheduling pattern across the same hours as traditional units. The pattern assures coverage for all days, 24-hours a day, 7 days a week, weekends or holidays. The cost of relief coverage is less overall, as many staff nurses work their off week to cover illness or vacations. As previously stated, the first 10 hours of work above the 7/70 schedule are straight time, so there is no overtime pay necessary. Additionally, department meetings, education, and

---

Box 2
Testimonials from the 7/70 registered nurse staff survey

"It is not just 7/70 itself that I like, but the no rotating of shifts and knowing what my work schedule is that I like even more!"

"Perhaps the greatest asset to a working mother is the gift of time. I feel 7/70 exemplifies this through its predictability that allows for such flexibility in both my career and personal life."

"Froedtert's 7/70 schedule has afforded me the opportunity to complete college courses and participate in advanced specialty courses related to my practice. I have also completed my medical–surgical nursing specialty certification. Additionally I have had the ability to chair the Nursing Development Council and attend related meetings and complete projects."

"Nurses love the consistency and time 7/70 allows; however, we especially love our 7 days off! Where else can you work full time and have 26 weeks off a year? 7/70 allows time for family, school, and much needed relaxation! Plus...what other hospital nurses can tell you they will be working Christmas Day in 2012?"

shared governance can all occur during overlap times, thereby eliminating added overtime. There is no need for agency or supplemental staffing. Recruitment costs are minimal, as word of mouth helps to recruit new graduates, who seem particularly interested in this staffing model as well as the expanded academic affiliations of the organization.

PATIENT SATISFACTION

Patient services offered at Froedtert Hospital include: cancer, neurosciences, trauma, transplant, cardiovascular, orthopedics, and women's health care. The organization is a certified adult rehabilitation facility and a Joint Commission-certified stroke center. The populations cared for are complex, and every nursing unit has telemetry capability. The added benefits of 7/70 for the patients are numerous. The actual and perceived continuity of care provided by the model is tremendously powerful as both a marketing and patient satisfaction tool. Having the same team caring for the patient every day provides a feeling of safety and comfort. Patients get to know their caregivers very well, and this creates a healing, caring bond that only enhances the patient experience within the relationship-centered model of care.

One patient described his experience in this manner,

"We appreciated the nursing scheduling, because it allowed us to get to know and count on the same professional nurse at the bedside every day for the 7 days. The nurses contributed to a sense of confidence about the quality of care we received at Froedtert and helped us to handle each stressful experience in the best way possible."

SUMMARY

The 7/70 scheduling and staffing pattern over the years has served Froedtert's nursing division and the patients very well. The hospital's registered nurse vacancy rate is consistently low, as is avoidable turnover. Registered nurse staff satisfaction is routinely validated with this model. New staff members are drawn to Froedtert Hospital by the unique, innovative, empowering scheduling plan. They often identify it and the academic relationships as the main reasons they choose to work at Froedtert Hospital. The predictability of schedules, the additional time provided by this 7/70 scheduling pattern allowing nurses to pursue professional growth, the overlap of staffing resources to assure quality care, and 26 scheduled weeks off a year give the nursing staff at Froedtert Hospital true respite from their workday stress. Through my work as a staff nurse using this model and later as the CNO, I felt I could be a personal and professional advocate for this model and my staff and for the patients through increased retention of experienced nurses.

REFERENCES

1. Leiter M, Jackson N, Shaughnessy K. Contrasting burnout, turnover, intention, control, value congruence, and knowledge sharing between baby boomers and generation X. J Nurs Manag 2009;17(1):100–9.
2. Buerhaus P, Donelan K, Ulrich B, et al. Registered nurse's perception of nursing. Nurs Econ 2005;23(3):110–8.
3. American Health Care Association Department of Research. Report of findings: 2007 AHCA survey nursing staff vacancy and turnover in nursing facilities.

Available at: http://www.ahcancal.org/research_data/staffing/Documents/Vacancy_Turnover_Survey2007.pdf. Accessed August 20, 2010.

4. Hendren R. Has the nursing shortage disappeared? Available at: http://www.healthleadersmedia.com/content/LED-254907/Has-the-Nursing-Shortage-Disappeared. Accessed August 10, 2010.

5. Jones C, Gates M. The costs and benefits of nurse turnover: a business case for nurse retention. Online J Issues Nurs. Available at: http://www.nursingworld.org/MainMenuCategories/ANAMarketplace/ANAPeriodicals/OJIN/TableofContents/Volume122007/No3Sept07/NurseRetention.aspx. Accessed August 20, 2010.

6. Leape L, Lawthers A, Brennan T, et al. Preventing medical injury. QRB Qual Rev Bull 1993;19(5):144–9.

Promoting Professional Nursing Practice: Linking a Professional Practice Model to Performance Expectations

Marcia Murphy, DNP, RN, ANP-BC[a],*, Barbara Hinch, DNP, RN, ACNP-BC[a],
Jane Llewellyn, PhD, RN, NEA-BC[b], Paula J. Dillon, MS, RN[c],
Elizabeth Carlson, PhD, RN[a]

KEYWORDS

- Professional practice model • Clinical advancement system
- Performance expectations • Magnet

Professional practice models (PPMs) provide a conceptual framework for establishing professional nursing practice. According to the American Nurses Credentialing Center's Magnet Recognition Program, a PPM is a schematic description of a system, theory, or phenomenon that depicts how nurses practice, collaborate, communicate, and develop to provide the highest quality of care for those served by the organization.[1,2] Integrating a PPM into the nursing practice arena may require complex organizational change. One strategy for integration is to directly link the PPM with performance expectations, thus ensuring that the underlying principles are supported and evident in everyday practice. This article describes the development, implementation, timeline, and successful outcomes of a clinical advancement system (CAS) that was aligned with a newly adopted PPM.

Rush University Medical Center (RUMC) is a tertiary-care academic medical center located in Chicago, Illinois, with more than 8000 employees. Each component of the four-part mission of the organization—patient care, research, education, and

This work was supported by Center for Clinical Research and Scholarship, Rush University Medical Center, Chicago, Illinois.
The authors have nothing to disclose.
[a] Department of Adult Health and Gerontological Nursing, Rush University College of Nursing, 600 South Paulina, Chicago, IL 60612, USA
[b] Rush University Medical Center, 1653 West Congress Parkway, 401 Jones, Chicago, IL 60612-3833, USA
[c] Department of Medical/Surgical Nursing, Rush University Medical Center, 1653 West Congress Parkway, 401 Jones, Chicago, IL 60612-3833, USA
* Corresponding author.
E-mail address: Marcia_murphy@rush.edu

Nurs Clin N Am 46 (2011) 67–79
doi:10.1016/j.cnur.2010.10.009
0029-6465/11/$ – see front matter © 2011 Published by Elsevier Inc.

community service—is driven by a focus on the provision of high-quality health care. The Division of Nursing at Rush has a long history of innovation, professional account-ability, and leadership in support of this mission. Innovations, including shared gover-nance, clinical advancement, and a practitioner-teacher model, were initially established in the 1970s and early 1980s. These structures have become embedded in the culture, beliefs, and practice of nursing and were evident when the organization received Magnet designation in 2002 and redesignation in 2006 and 2010.

RUMC nursing leadership spearheaded the development and adoption of a PPM in 2005 to promote continued advancement of professional nursing practice within the system. A comprehensive process was undertaken to develop The Rush Model of Professional Nursing Practice. The model is consistent with the mission, vision, and values of RUMC while integrating key beliefs and practices set forth in nursing's mission and philosophy. **Table 1** illustrates the alignment and integration of the Rush Model within the medical center.

The Rush Model describes the concepts of relationships and caring as the basis for nursing practice at RUMC (**Fig. 1**). This is depicted in the outer circle of the model. Nursing practice exists within the caring, therapeutic relationship between the nurse and the patient/family. The Rush Model identifies key characteristics of the nurse-patient relationship, which include collaboration, intentional presence, cultural sensi-tivity, compassion, and respect. The model also depicts three intertwining circles that represent the primary domains of skill that the professional nurse integrates to meet the needs of patients and families. These skills include critical thinking, application of evidence-based interventions, and technical expertise. As these three domains develop within each nurse's individual practice, leadership skills begin to emerge. Leadership takes shape in each situation in which the nurse practices and differs in scope by nursing position.

INTEGRATING PROFESSIONAL PRACTICE MODELS

Many organizations are at some phase of the Magnet journey and are, therefore, inter-ested in the development of a PPM for nursing. The Magnet Recognition Program identifies a PPM as an overarching conceptual framework for nurses, nursing care, and interdisciplinary patient care. The alignment of nursing performance expectations with the PPM has been one strategy for adoption. At Strong Memorial Hospital, a PPM was developed to support the mission, vision, and values of the institution and is evident in daily work.[3] This model was used to develop nursing job descriptions and performance evaluation mechanisms. The key concepts of caring services, discov-ering new knowledge, teaching others, and continuous learning were used as common threads in the development of the model, job descriptions, and evaluation methods. Vanderbilt University Medical Center developed a performance-based career advancement system based on the Vanderbilt Professional Nursing Practice Model and Benner's model for developing clinical excellence.[4,5] The practice model includes six key functions for the nurse—planning and managing care, care planning, education, communication, collaboration, and continuous learning—and has been successfully implemented in a variety of practice settings.[4]

Clarian Health Partners in Indianapolis adopted the American Association of Critical-Care Nurses Synergy Model for Patient Care to guide their process toward Magnet recognition.[6] This model includes three components: nurse competency, patient char-acteristics, and the organization. The eight competencies for professional nursing practice in the model serve as the infrastructure for the professional advancement process. Titles for professional nurses in this system are associate partner, partner,

Table 1
Linkage between CAS and RUMC's mission, vision, and values

RUMC Mission, Vision, and Values	Division of Nursing Mission and Vision	RUMC Model of Professional Nursing Practice	Accountable Professional Nursing Practice	Patient/Family Outcomes

• Innovation
• Collaboration
• Accountability
• Respect
• Excellence
	Rush nurses
	Respond to cultural differences
	Use evidence-based practice
	Support family centered care
	Help patients move through a continuum of care
	PNS goals
	• To promote a high level of professional performance among professional nurses
		• Relationships and caring
		  Care is patient/family centered
		  Respect
		  Collaborative practice
		• Critical thinking
		  Reasoned clinical judgment
		  Applies science
		• Technical expertise
		  Patient safety
		  Patient education
		• Application of evidence-based interventions
		  Interventions based on research
		  Standards of care reflect current research
		• Leadership
		  Accountability
		  Continuous learning
			Rush clinical advancement system	• Satisfaction with care
				• Quality care
				• Safety
				
				Nursing staff
				• Job satisfaction
				• Retention
				• Career Progression
				• Scholarly activities
				  Organizational outcomes
				• Foundational values evident in everyday practice of professional nurses

Illustrates the integration of the RUMC model of professional nursing practice within the medical center. Column 1 describes RUMC's core values. Column 2 represents an excerpt from the Division of Nursing mission and vision, along with the shared governance model goals. Column 3 describes the domains of the PPM. Column 4 identifies practice and the CAS as primary outcomes. Columns 1–4 influence significant medical center outcomes, which are listed in column 5.

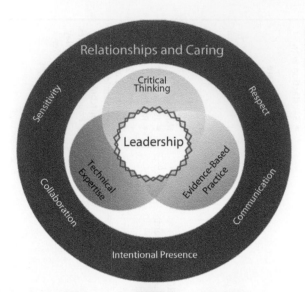

Relationships and Caring
•Care is patient and family centered
•Respect
•Collaborative practice
•Sensitivity to diversity and culture

Critical Thinking
•Reasoned clinical judgment
•Applies science

Technical Expertise
•Patient safety
•Patient education

Evidence-Based Practice
•Interventions based on research
•Standards of care reflect current practice

Leadership
•Accountability
•Continuous learning

RUSH UNIVERSITY MEDICAL CENTER CLINICAL ADVANCEMENT SYSTEM
RNI
RNII
RNIII
CNC

Fig. 1. The Rush Model of Professional Nursing Practice. This figure is a pictorial representation of The Rush Model of Professional Nursing Practice. The primary domains of the model are listed along with key aspects within each domain. The arrow depicts the alignment of the PPM with the clinical advancement system.

and senior partner. Partners must hold specialty certification and senior partners must hold a baccalaureate degree, thus supporting professional advancement. Clarian has used the synergy model to measure outcomes. Vacancy and turnover rates have decreased and nurse, patient, and family satisfaction has improved.[5] In addition, the number of nurses with specialty certification increased from 15% to 40%.

Holy Cross Hospital in Maryland integrated the quality care model into the design of a care delivery system.[7] The registered nurse (RN) job description was revised to reflect the model, including the development of desired behaviors and competencies.

This system identified the importance of leadership development, staff education in the implementation of a PPM, and inclusion of the director of human resources (HR) as a key stakeholder.

PROCESS AND TIME FRAMES AT RUMC

The first step in the integration of The Rush Model of Professional Nursing Practice at RUMC was the redesign of the CAS. Although the CAS was well established and had been in place since the 1970s, it had not been updated for 12 years. This system included three clinical levels and a clinical leadership role, providing career advancement for Rush nurses. Performance expectations were defined for each level as well as within position descriptions. In 2006, however, it was recognized that the previous system did not integrate and support the newly adopted PPM. Two project directors were appointed to lead the project with the goals of (1) aligning performance expectations with the new PPM and (2) updating the clinical advancement. The overall process began the summer of 2006 and culminated in the rollout of the new CAS in September of 2008.

The Kellogg Foundation Logic Model Development Guide[8] was used as the framework for change, including program planning, implementation, and evaluation. This process began with a well-defined problem and basic assumptions. The assumptions were (1) nursing at RUMC has a history of leadership, innovation, and professional accountability; (2) the Illinois Nurse Practice Act, American Nurses Association Social Policy Statement, and American Nurses Association Code of Ethics guide professional nursing practice; (3) a PPM drives role responsibilities as defined by position descriptions; (4) the professional nurse directs care as part of a health care team; unlicensed, assistive personnel are part of the team; (5) seasoned, experienced nurses possess intellectual capital that is valued by the organization; (6) baccalaureate-prepared nurses possess the scientific and theoretic knowledge base to meet the complex needs of patients and families; and (7) national certification demonstrates that an individual has mastered a body of knowledge and acquired skills in a particular specialty. These assumptions served to guide the development of project objectives, activities, and outcome evaluation plan.

The initial phase (summer of 2006) of this process was to obtain input and support for the project from key stakeholders in the organization, including the vice president of nursing, nursing directors and unit directors, executive committee of the professional nursing staff (PNS), vice president of HR, and the Magnet coordinator. The executive committee of PNS is the leadership group of the shared governance model and is composed of staff nurses representing the various specialties in the medical center. A PowerPoint presentation was developed to describe the problem statement, assumptions, goals, activities, timeline, outcomes, and impact to solicit input as well as to gain support from the key stakeholders of this project. This inclusive, collegial process engaged stakeholders in the development of the project plan. These key stakeholders enthusiastically provided support for this project, which was important to secure the necessary resources to accomplish the project goals. It was also important to establish the foundation for the future sustainability of this project.

The next phase (fall of 2006) of the project was to use a focus group format to solicit input from nursing staff regarding their current role responsibilities. This was the initial step of a comprehensive process to develop and validate competencies per level to gain a better understanding of current role responsibilities across all levels of staff. In addition, this approach facilitated the direct involvement of nurses in this major change initiative. Unit leadership invited staff nurses to volunteer to participate in this process. Twelve focus groups were conducted with 7 to 10 nurses in each group representing the various departments within the Division of Nursing. The groups were homogeneous in terms of level within the current advancement system. More than 100 professional nurses participated in this process. An additional focus group was held, which was composed of unit directors representing the various departments.

The focus groups were planned carefully. Three components define successful focus groups: a well-defined purpose, carefully planned environment, and skilled facilitator.[9] The groups had a clearly defined purpose. Convenient, comfortable conference rooms were identified for the focus groups. Scheduling included consideration of staff working all shifts and weekends.

Open-ended questions were developed to solicit staff nurse perspectives regarding their current practice based on the domains of the Rush PPM. Two facilitators were present during the sessions. One facilitator led the discussion while the second took detailed minutes. The focus groups were taped. Written, informed consent permitting the taping of the session was obtained from each participant. Internal review board approval was secured.

The next phase of activities (January through May of 2007) was to write the first draft of the PNS position descriptions. The comprehensive qualitative data from the focus groups served as an analysis of current nursing responsibilities. A job analysis is a systematic way of gathering information about the content, context, and human requirements of jobs.[10] The minutes and tapes from the focus groups were analyzed. The data were coded and synthesized to identify themes, which were used in the development of the first draft of the redesigned position descriptions.

Benner's model[5] was used as the theoretic framework to define clinical advancement. Several organizations have used this model to guide the development of their CAS successfully.[4,11] A summary profile was written to clearly differentiate practice levels and guide the development of competencies within each specific position description (**Box 1**).

The competencies within the position descriptions were organized based on the domains of the Rush model of professional nursing practice. These domains include critical thinking, evidence-based interventions, technical expertise, leadership, relationships, and caring. Competencies per level were written based on the job analysis data. In addition, key documents were also analyzed and synthesized into the development. These documents included Illinois Nurse Practice Act; PNS bylaws; organization's mission, vision, and values; and national safety goals. This process culminated in the development of three clinical advancement levels and a clinical leadership role. An example of the leadership domain is shown in **Table 2**.

The next phase (May through July of 2007) of project activities focused on validation of the draft position descriptions, which included an expert panel review and pilot study. A review of the nursing literature did not reveal an example of validation of competencies within CASs. Because of the scope of this change, it was considered essential that validation of position descriptions occurred before transitioning more than 1000 staff nurses into the new system.

An expert panel review was used to establish content validity.[12] The expert panel included staff nurses representing the five departments, unit directors, and departmental director. The group achieved consensus on the appropriate level for each specific competency. Each competency was examined for clarity and relevance for current practice. Minor revisions were made in the first draft of the position descriptions based on the input from this expert panel.

A pilot study was conducted in June of 2007 on five units representing the various departments in the Division of Nursing. The purpose was to determine content validity

---

Box 1
Clinical advancement system levels

RN1

The novice is a beginning level nurse. Uses scientific and theoretic knowledge base along with policy and procedures, standards of care, and protocols to guide practice. Relies on the experience judgment and support of others while developing knowledge in practice. Words/ phrases characteristic of this level: beginning, seeks appropriate information, with guidance.

RN2

The competent nurse has mastered the technical skills. Is aware of patterns of patient responses and can use past experiences to identify solutions for current situations. Continues to consult other members of the health care team when the need for assistance is identified. Word/ phrases characteristic of this level: consistent, prioritize care activities, able to individualize care.

RN3

Proficient nurses have an in-depth knowledge of patient management. Can accommodate unplanned events and can respond with efficiency, flexibility, and confidence. Immediately sees the whole situation while being able to discriminate what is most relevant. Has developed advanced communication and collaboration skills along with system savvy. Assumes a leadership role in the clinical practice area, using clinical experience to serve as a role model and coach. Words/phrases characteristic of this level: advanced, role model, resource, critically analyzes, anticipates.

Clinical nurse coordinator (CNC)

Experienced nurse with the responsibility and accountability for nursing practice as delegated by unit director. Provides leadership for nursing staff in collaboration with unit director.

---

and to determine whether or not the position descriptions accurately reflected practice at each level. Two staff nurses were randomly selected from each level to participate with a total of 38 nurses participating in the pilot study. Each nurse completed a log at the end of each shift for 2 weeks, which included competencies from the draft position descriptions. Staff were asked to check the competencies that they performed during each shift. They were also asked to respond to two open-ended questions: (1) Which of the above competencies that you did not perform today would you consider important if you had the opportunity? (2) What did you do today that was not captured in the above competencies?

Overall, 80% of the competencies for the RN1 position were validated, 85% of the competencies were validated for the RN2 position, 75% for the RN3 position, and 64% for the CNC position were validated. A detailed analysis of the data influenced some revisions in the position descriptions. For example, the nurses who completed the log sheets in the CNC level identified that direct patient management was not adequately represented in the log. Therefore, revisions were made in the position description. Two competencies were added that reflect the direct management of patients.

Unit directors on these units also participated in this pilot study. The unit director completed an evaluation of a randomly selected staff nurse from each level. The evaluation tool was comprised of the competencies within the draft position descriptions. In addition, the managers were to respond to several open-ended questions. The overall proportion of statements validated for the RN1 position was 75%, RN2 position was 80%, RN3 position was 75%, and CNC position was 95%. Overall, the unit directors commented that the draft position descriptions differentiated practice accurately at each level and that the competencies were clear and measurable. No revisions were

Table 2 Leadership domain			
RN 1	**RN 2**	**RN 3**	**CNC**
Supports unit goals and change initiatives	Demonstrates the ability to effectively precept staff and students on the unit	Serves as a role model whose beliefs, attitudes, and actions support unit leadership and unit goals	Assumes the accountability of administrative functions of the unit as delegated by the unit director
Demonstrates beginning delegation skills to meet the needs of patients	Demonstrates beginning leadership skills related to patient care	Demonstrates proficient leadership skills at the unit level	Functions as a mentor to staff on the unit
Demonstrates accountability for own professional practice, including progress toward achievement of annual goals	Delegates effectively and consistently to optimize patient outcomes	Demonstrates accountability for own professional practice, including progress toward achievement of annual goals	Assumes a leadership role in analytical problem solving of both clinical and system wide issues
	Demonstrates accountability for own professional practice, including progress toward achievement of annual goals		Demonstrates accountability for own professional practice, including progress toward achievement of annual goals

made in the position descriptions based on the analysis of the data from the unit directors. This pilot study along with the expert panel review culminated in a CAS with validated and feasible performance expectations.

During August and September of 2007, the project was presented again to key stakeholders to communicate project results, solicit input, and gain support. The response from the various groups to the presentation was positive and, ultimately, the new CAS was formally approved by Nursing Operations Council in October of 2007.

IMPLEMENTATION

An implementation task force was established in January of 2008. The goals of this group were to design and implement a strategy and process to transition all professional nurses into the new CAS. The transition of more than 1000 nurses was a substantial undertaking mandating a comprehensive, well-designed plan. The task force developed a timeline for their work. Employee evaluations based on the established position descriptions were conducted in July and August in anticipation of the transition to the new CAS in September of 2008. This timeline served as a useful tool to track the progress of the group work.

At the initial meeting, the task force members reviewed the performance expectations across the levels in the new CAS. The expectations were intentionally written in a general, rather than detailed, manner. This is consistent with typical position description format developed by HR.[10] Position descriptions written in this format allow for applicability across specialties and areas of practice.

The ultimate goal of the new CAS was to redefine practice at all levels of staff so that it would consistently reflect the PPM. Therefore, the task force thought that it was essential that staff and managers have "a clear picture of practice" at each level to gain an understanding of the new performance expectations. It was decided that it would be useful for staff and managers to have specific behavioral activities reflecting each expectation. The group decided that focus groups of nursing staff would be an effective way to develop these specific behaviors.[4]

At RUMC, the project directors conducted four focus groups. The groups represented each level in the current system and the various specialties across the medical center. The primary question posed to each group was, How would you demonstrate that you were meeting the performance expectations within this newly developed position description? The staff within each focus group developed a list of relevant, realistic behaviors that would serve to highlight the change in practice competencies at each level. This document later served as a key educational tool for all nursing staff and managers across the medical center. **Box 2** provides an example of these activities in the leadership domain for the RN2 position.

The next major task was to develop a toolkit for each unit to aid in implementation. The contents of the toolkit included a letter from the vice president of nursing, the Rush PPM, the new CAS position descriptions, examples of specific behavioral activities to meet the competencies within each position description, a case study illustrating the nursing care interventions at each level, frequently asked questions, specific transition guidelines, and information regarding certification. Therefore, this comprehensive

---

Box 2
Sample behavior activities for RN2 leadership domain

Demonstrates the ability to effectively precept staff and students on the unit
- Monitors progress of new staff in meeting orientation goals along with unit leadership
- Collaborates with nursing instructors regarding student performance

Demonstrates beginning leadership skills related to patient care
- Functions as an effective charge nurse
- Participates in the staffing process of the department on a regular basis, including matching the competency of the nurse with the needs of patients
- Demonstrates accountability to ensure quality patient outcomes (monitors self and others)
- Use system resources in problem solving patient care situations
- Communicates issues to management that require additional follow-up

Delegates effectively and consistently to optimize patient outcomes
- Delegating patient assignments as charge nurse
- Demonstrates consistent and effective delegation to patient care technicians and other unit personnel

Demonstrates accountability for own professional practice, including progress toward achievement of annual goals
- Responsible for self-evaluation, maintains portfolio
- Takes advantage of learning opportunities throughout the medical center
- Presents in-services on unit
- Identifies professional goals

resource included information that addressed the commonly asked questions as well as implications regarding the transition to the new system as it was introduced on the unit level.

The educational and marketing plan included face-to-face sessions along with the toolkit and posters for each unit depicting the alignment of the new CAS with the PPM. Thirteen information sessions held on all shifts and weekends were conducted for staff nurses across the medical center. A goal of these sessions was to share the background, development, transitions guidelines, and expected outcomes of the new CAS. The focus of the questions from the staff revolved around the qualifications designated for each position. One concern that consistently arose was the lack of reimbursement by the medical center for part-time staff to pursue programs, such as certification review courses. A representative from HR was present at each session, who helped respond to questions and noted the theme regarding lack of financial support for part-time staff. Nursing leadership developed a proposal requesting a change in the corporation's reimbursement policies for part-time benefited employees. This proposal was submitted and, ultimately, HR was able to secure funds in their budget to support part-time staff's pursuit of educational offerings and certification.

Similar educational sessions were held for all unit managers. This group was the key stakeholder group to reinforce the new performance expectations throughout the year. Also, this group would be conducting the performance evaluations based on the new position descriptions so it was important to ensure consistency.

COLLABORATION WITH HUMAN RESOURCES

A subgroup of the implementation task force met with key representatives from HR. The nursing director was a key member of this group because of her in-depth, comprehensive knowledge of medical center operations. Three HR representatives were part of this group, including the director of HR. This type of initiative mandates effective collaboration with HR.[7] The initial meeting with HR focused on establishing guiding principles for this planning process. These principles included the following: the transition process to the new position descriptions will be conducted consistent with the Rush values, the salary structure remains the same, the number of clinical levels remains the same, and evaluations in summer of 2008 will be conducted according to current policy and the current position descriptions. This collaborative effort focused on developing specific transition guidelines. These guidelines addressed all levels and categories of staff across the medical center.

Additional work included formatting the new position descriptions into the standard HR format and the determination of qualifications per level. The new CAS differentiated practice at each level by advancing performance expectations. These expectations were achievable based on the development of an individual nurse's knowledge and skills within the domains of practice: relationships and caring, critical thinking evidenced-based interventions, technical expertise, and leadership. This new system posed the opportunity to establish qualifications necessary for consideration of promotion to the next level. The nursing director member of the implementation task force led discussions within the nursing leadership group regarding this. The initial project assumptions guided this process. Also, the strategic plan, which included a goal to increase the percentage of baccalaureate-prepared nurses, influenced this decision making. The vision and goals were considered along with practical recruitment issues in certain areas. The outcome of these discussions culminated in the qualifications depicted in **Box 3**.

Box 3
Qualifications for position descriptions

RN1

1. Baccalaureate degree in nursing or other major

2. Associate degree prepared nurse enrolled in a bachelor of science in nursing program, baccalaureate program, or master's in nursing program

RN2

1. Consistent proficient performance at RN1 position or equivalent experience

2. Baccalaureate degree in nursing or other major

RN3

1. Consistent proficient performance at RN2 position or equivalent experience

2. Baccalaureate degree in nursing or other major

3. National certification

CNC

1. Consistent proficient performance at the RN3 level or equivalent experience

2. Demonstrated progressive, proficient management and leadership skills

3. Baccalaureate degree in nursing or other major

4. National certification

OUTCOMES

A comprehensive outcome evaluation plan was developed in the following domains: turnover, professional practice, and satisfaction, with turnover identified as the key outcome of this project. The rollout of this new system represented a transformational change in roles and expectations for professional nurses. Moreover, the new qualifications had an impact on many practicing nurses who would be required to obtain a baccalaureate degree and/or certification. Therefore, the impact of the new CAS on turnover was important to evaluate. The overall turnover before implementation was 14.25%. One year after implementation, the turnover was 9.3%. Although many factors influenced this drop in turnover, including the economy, this outcome indicated a successful transition to the new CAS.

The outcomes related to professional practice included the percentage of staff with baccalaureate degrees and certifications. It was expected that the new qualifications would influence an increase in both categories. The percentage of nurses with baccalaureate degrees increased from 80% in 2008 to 83% in 2009, 1 year post implementation. The expectation is that this percentage will continue to increase. There was a substantial increase in the percentage of staff nurses with certifications. The number of newly certified nurses has nearly doubled, increasing from 55 new certifications in 2008 to 108 new certifications in 2009.

A survey was developed to determine both staff nurse and manager satisfaction with the newly adopted CAS. Content validity was established by a panel of three experts, including nursing leadership and a qualitative researcher.[12] Institutional review board approval was obtained before distribution of the survey. Sixty-eight surveys were sent via email to all unit directors and CNCs. Fifty surveys (74% response rate) were realized. Approximately 35% of staff nurses within each level

Table 3
Satisfaction survey results percentage of respondents who agree or strongly agree to this shaded area

Survey Question	Staff (n = 64)	Managers (n = 50)
The position descriptions reflect the PPM of the Division of Nursing at RUMC	95%	96%
The position descriptions reflect the values of RUMC	95%	96%
The position descriptions provide a mechanism for career advancement for nurses at RUMC	84%	92%
The position descriptions clearly differentiate practice at each level	84%	90%
The competencies within each position description are clearly worded	78%	86%
The competencies within each position description are attainable	87%	94%
The position descriptions capture all competencies necessary for practice within my/each level	85%	82%
I am satisfied with the new clinical advancement system	79%	85%
I know what is expected of me to advance to the next level (staff only)	80%	—
I am able to effectively evaluate my staff with the new position descriptions (managers only)	—	83%

were selected to receive the survey. A total of 350 surveys were sent to staff nurses. Sixty-four staff nurse surveys were returned (18% response rate), which is an 18% response. Several factors may have influenced this low response, including several new hospital initiatives, concurrent surveys, and annual employee evaluation time in the medical center.

The results of the staff and manager surveys are displayed in **Table 3**. Overall, the results are positive, with at least 78% of respondents agreeing and strongly agreeing on all survey items. Also, both staff nurses and managers are satisfied with the new CAS. The low staff response rate presents a limitation to this survey analysis.

SUMMARY

The process of aligning a PPM with performance expectations demanded a commitment of time and effort on the part of leadership and staff nurses. The transition at RUMC represents a transformational change because role responsibilities were redefined for more than 1000 nurses. There were several strategies that promoted the success of this project. First, a prerequisite to this initiative was a clearly articulated leadership vision. Additionally, a mature shared governance model promoted a commitment to continued advancement as well as innovation. Stakeholder support and involvement throughout the process promoted effective integration into medical center operations. Furthermore, 160 professional nurses and managers were directly involved in this process at some level. This grass roots approach facilitated successful implementation and transition of the CAS at RUMC and support the Magnet culture of excellence.

ACKNOWLEDGMENTS

Ruth Kleinpell, PhD, RN, FAAN, for editorial assistance and support. Rose Suhayda, PhD, RN, for assistance with survey development and data analysis.

REFERENCES

1. American Nurses Association. ANCC Magnet recognition program recognition excellence in nursing services. American Nurses Credentialing Center. Available at: www.nursecredentialing.org/magnet.aspx. Accessed August 24, 2010.
2. Storey S, Linden E, Fisher M. Showcasing leadership exemplars to propel professional practice model implementation. J Nurs Adm 2010;3(3):138–42.
3. Ingersoll G, Witzel P, Smith T. Using organizational mission, vision and values to guide professional practice model development and measurement of nurse performance. J Nurs Adm 2005;35(2):86–93.
4. Robinson K, Eck C, Keck B, et al. The Vanderbilt professional practice program. Part 1: growing and supporting professional nursing practice. J Nurs Adm 2003; 33(9):441–50.
5. Benner P. From novice to expert: excellence and power in clinical nursing practice. Menlo Park (CA): Addison-Wesley; 1984.
6. Kerfoot K, Lavandero R, Cox M, et al. Conceptual models and the nursing organization: implementing the AACN synergy model for patient care. Nurse Leader 2006;4(4):20–6.
7. Duffy J, Baldwin J, Mastorovich MJ. Using the quality-caring model to organize patient care delivery. J Nurs Adm 2007;37(12):546–51.
8. W.K. Kellogg foundation logic model development guide. Battle Creek (MI): W.K. Kellogg Foundation; 2004. 15–25.
9. Cote-Arsenault D, Morrison-Beedy D. Maintaining your focus in focus groups: avoiding common mistakes. Res Nurs Health 2005;28:172–9.
10. Mathis R, Jackson J. Jobs and job analysis. In: Human resource management. 12th edition. Mason (OH): Thomson South-Western; 2008. p. 160–90.
11. Krugman M, Smith K, Goode C. A clinical advancement program; evaluating 10 years of progressive change. J Nurs Adm 2000;35(2):86–93.
12. Polit D, Beck CT. Assessing measurement quality in quantitative studies. In: Nursing research: generating and assessing evidence for nursing practice. 8th edition. Philadelphia: Wolters Kluwer, Lipincott Williams & Wilkins; 2008. p. 458–9.

Building an Engaged and Certified Nursing Workforce

Dale Callicutt, MSN, RN-BC, CCRN[a,b,c,d,*],
Karen Norman, MSN, RN-BC, CCRN[a,c], Lesa Smith, MSN, RN-BC, CCRN[a,c],
Audrey Nichols, RN-BC[a], Daria Kring, PhD, RN-BC[a]

KEYWORDS

- Certification • Employee engagement • Magnet

Professional certification has been linked to positive patient, system, and nurse outcomes. However, certification rates among nurses remain low. The purpose of this initiative was to improve the certification rates of our cardiac nursing staff. Using tenets from employee engagement theory, we designed strategies to fully engage nurses within our nursing division to pursue certification. After 1 year, certification rates more than doubled in our cardiac departments.

IMPORTANCE OF CERTIFICATION

Certification is achieved when "a nongovernmental agency or association certifies that an individual licensed to practice a profession has met certain predetermined standards specified by that profession for specialty practice."[1] The American Nurses Credentialing Center (ANCC) and other nursing specialty organizations are the agencies within the profession of nursing that determine the scope of nursing specialty practice, design measurement criteria for assessing mastery of knowledge, and convey the rights to use specific credentials as an indication of successful certification. The American Nurses Association began certifying nurses in the 1970s exclusively for professional acknowledgment.[2] Today, certification confirms a nurse's attainment of a specific, specialty-related body of knowledge.

The authors have nothing to disclose.
[a] Forsyth Medical Center, 3333 Silas Creek Parkway, Winston-Salem, NC 27103, USA
[b] Cardiac-Vascular Nurse Content Expert Panel, ANCC, 8515 Georgia Avenue, Suite 400, Silver Springs, MA 20910–3492, USA
[c] Winston-Salem State University, 601 South Martin Luther King Jr Drive, Winston-Salem, NC 27110, USA
[d] University of North Carolina at Greensboro, 1400 Spring Garden Street, Greensboro, NC 27412, USA
* Corresponding author. Forsyth Medical Center, 3333 Silas Creek Parkway, Winston-Salem, North Carolina 27103.
E-mail address: jdcallicutt@novanthealth.org

Nurs Clin N Am 46 (2011) 81–87
doi:10.1016/j.cnur.2010.10.004
0029-6465/11/$ – see front matter © 2011 Elsevier Inc. All rights reserved.

Certification is more than the passage of an examination. Research is beginning to show that certified nurses contribute to better patient, system, and nursing outcomes. Cary[3] found that certified nurses have a direct link to lower patient mortalities and higher patient satisfaction. Another study found that the proportion of certified staff was inversely related to patient falls.[4] Fitzpatrick and colleagues[5] reported that certified critical care nurses have higher levels of empowerment and are less likely to leave the profession than their noncertified colleagues. Finally, Craven[6] investigated a medical-surgical unit with a high percentage of certified nurses and reported a low vacancy rate and high patient satisfaction.

Nursing certification is not only important within the profession, but also within the community. The conscientious health care consumer is often knowledgeable about the meaning of certification. In fact, a poll conducted by the American Association of Critical-Care Nurses found that 78% of consumers knew about nursing certification and 73% stated they prefer a hospital that employs certified nurses.[7] Consumers expect expert knowledge and understand that certification is a way to validate this knowledge.[7]

Other health professionals also use a certification process to demonstrate the attainment of specialty knowledge. In truth, certification is more of an expectation for our physician colleagues. Ninety percent of physicians are board certified by their respective specialty organizations.[2] However, Magnet hospitals, for which nursing certification is a required benchmark, report a mean certification rate of only 27.6%, according to statistics presented at the ANCC National Magnet Conference in 2009. Nonmagnet hospitals often have much lower certification rates. The reasons for this underachievement have been well documented. Nurses report that they avoid certification because of costs associated with study materials and examination fees, fear associated with not passing the examination, lack of recognition by their organization for achieving certification, and inconsequential professional benefits.[8]

Given the evidence in support of nursing certification, and the lack of nurses actively pursuing certification, the challenge for magnet hospitals becomes finding ways to increase percentages of nurses with specialty certification. For our organization, the answer was embedded in employee engagement theory.

EMPLOYEE ENGAGEMENT

Employee engagement is simply defined as "a person who is fully involved in, and enthusiastic about, his or her work."[9] Rutledge[10] describes the engaged employee as one who is not only attracted to his or her work, but inspired by it, committed to it, and fascinated by it. However, engagement does not only benefit the employee. Organizations with engaged workforces are 56% more likely to have above-average customer loyalty and 27% more likely to have higher profitability.[11] In addition, engaged employees are 20% more likely to perform better and 87% less likely to leave the organization.[11]

Engagement occurs in 2 distinct dimensions.[12–14] One dimension is rational, which is the commitment of the mind. This develops when the employee benefits financially, professionally, and developmentally from his or her teams, leader, and organization. The other dimension is emotional, which is commitment of the heart. Emotional commitment is believing, valuing, or enjoying the day-to-day activities, work teams, leadership, and organization as a whole.

Although many managers believe that extrinsic factors, such as salary, contribute significantly to employee engagement, there is little evidence to support this. In contrast, there are at least 5 intrinsic motivators that create engagement[15]: being in healthy relationships with others, having meaningful work, progressing with one's work, having choices, and being involved in decision making. When these motivators are in place, employees are much more likely to be engaged in the workplace. Similarly, Maslach and colleagues[16] identified 6 areas of work life that enhance engagement: manageable workload, control over work, rewards and recognition, community and social support, perceived fairness, and congruent values. Seijts and Crim[9] summarized the engagement literature into the 10 C's of employee engagement. According to their framework, leaders wanting to engage their employees should reach out and Connect with them, provide opportunities for Career advancement, provide a Clear vision, Convey meaningful feedback, Congratulate strong performance, allow for employee Contributions and Control over their work, encourage Collaboration among team members, establish Credible standards, and create Confidence.

PURPOSE

The leadership team of our cardiac services division wanted to improve the certification rate in our division. Having achieved magnet designation and redesignation 4 years later, we were proud of the important part that certified nurses played in reaching that goal. We also knew that to remain an exemplary organization, we would need to continue to improve this important metric. In 2009, our cardiac services division had 6% certified staff in the telemetry areas, and 13% certified staff in the critical care area. Our stretch goal was to double these statistics within 1 year.

A couple of years before this initiative, a national expert was brought in to teach a certification review course for the ANCC Cardiac Vascular Nurse certification examination. This endeavor produced a minimal number of certified nurses. Simply setting the expectation that nurses will become certified had little impact on motivating staff. Indeed, our most engaged staff had already achieved certification. We now needed to reach out to staff who were much more reluctant to take this professional step. We turned to employee engagement theory.

Using a mixture of engagement tenets set forth by organizational experts, we identified a framework in which to develop specific strategies to increase certification rates. This framework, supported by evidence from the employee engagement literature, consisted of

1. Establishing greater meaning to work
2. Communicating a shared vision
3. Encouraging decision making
4. Creating a sense of team
5. Enhancing career opportunities
6. Rewarding success.

METHODS

Using the 6 engagement tenets, our leadership team developed specific strategies to transform our division by highly engaging our employees through the certification process. To establish greater meaning to our work (tenet #1), leaders began the certification project by imparting inspiration. Our initial information sessions did not focus as much on the logistics of certification, but rather on how certification can transform a clinical department. Certification bolsters collegial relationships because it acknowledges to others the achievement of specialty knowledge that is associated with proficient skill performance and favorable patient outcomes. We stressed that demonstrating this knowledge through specialty certification allows nurses to tangibly document the quality care they provide. It is one thing to intuitively believe you have attained proficient knowledge, it is quite another to have empirical evidence of that knowledge. Once achieved, certification brings a sense of accomplishment that reaches beyond daily care—it validates years of meaningful work in one specialty area.

To effectively engage nurses in the certification project, the leaders realized that communicating our shared vision of certification (tenet #2) was important. Leaders from every cardiac department stepped forward to promote certification. They set a clear vision that cardiac services would lead the organization in nursing certification. This call to action was noticed by staff from both within and outside cardiac services. To further demonstrate the value placed on certification, the leaders agreed to pay for certification examinations up front, with no payback requirement. For many nurses, the high degree of value placed on certification by their leader moved them from noncommittal to full engagement in the process.

To encourage staff decision making (tenet #3), leaders designed the certification initiative in collaboration with staff nurses. Several nurses stepped forward to drive the project in their particular work area. Tapping into the energy and knowledge of these key staff nurses, the leadership team held planning meetings to create a challenging yet doable strategy for certification readiness. This strategy included staff-led study groups, didactic review classes, e-mailed review questions, and case study discussions. Efforts were made to support and encourage nurses in multiple ways to study and prepare for certification. All the approaches were designed with staff nurse input to ensure feasibility, garner support, and foster continued engagement. For example, study groups were held at convenient times for nurses to work with peers, and review courses were taught by certified nurses within the organization as well as by national speakers.

Even with the emerging culture change within our division, many nurses were apprehensive about the certification process. From nurses who had only a couple of years of tenure in the specialty, to nurses who had been out of school for many years, the requirement of testing one's knowledge was daunting. To engage these nurses, we created a sense of team (tenet #4). Study groups were formed in the telemetry departments around working schedules, which meant staff studied with their coworkers. Rather than foster a sense of competition among individuals (who can get certified first?), the focus was on group learning and mutual support. Each cohort had a staff nurse leader who ensured the study group remained team-focused. The teams went through the core curriculum as a group, allowing study sessions to be a safe and comfortable place to ask questions and seek clarity about complex clinical concepts. As the weeks progressed, the teams became close-knit groups with highly engaged team members. Even when other commitments threatened attendance, no one dropped out of the groups because the support was genuine, confidence was bolstered, and nurses were proud to be part of a select group that was studying for certification.

Engaged employees are high performers because they see the opportunities awaiting them in the organization (tenet #5). With no growth opportunities, employees often become bored and apathetic. Nursing is certainly a career at risk for stagnation. To engage our nurses who did not see the personal growth benefit of certification, we implemented personal career counseling. Leaders designed a process for quarterly one-on-one sessions with staff nurses to determine career goals as well as academic and professional opportunities needed to reach those goals. These career roadmaps almost always recommended professional certification. Whether the nurse wanted to move into administration or grow in place as an expert practitioner, certification was endorsed as a career-enhancing and valued accomplishment by nursing leaders. By understanding the competitive edge that certification can provide, nurses became more engaged in valuing it for their personal career goals.

Finally, the certification initiative rewarded nurses in several ways for successfully achieving certification (tenet #6). Banners were posted on the unit when each nurse passed the examination and a notification was sent to all members of the department and leadership via e-mail. Leaders sent congratulation notes to newly certified nurses. Nurses placed their new certification credentials on their name badge and their certification certificate was displayed on the unit's Wall of Honor. All newly certified nurses were listed by name in the hospital's annual nursing report, which was distributed to all nurses and organization leaders. Certified nurses were invited to an annual celebration during National Nurse Certification Day in March. In addition, certification counts toward the career ladder program that monetarily compensates nurses for demonstrated excellence in clinical and professional activities. Nurses achieving career ladder promotion were listed on unit plaques.

RESULTS

After 1 year of implementing specific and intentional strategies to enhance employee engagement around certification, we have seen improvements in our certification rates for every cardiac department. In the critical care areas, of the 82 eligible nurses, 30 have achieved certification; thereby raising the rate from 13% to 37%, more than exceeding our goal to double the rate. In the telemetry unit, of the 99 eligible nurses, 28 have attained certification. This achievement raised our certification percentage from 6% to 28%—a fourfold increase. As the project gained momentum, other cardiac areas wanted to participate. The cardiac procedural and outpatient areas had 12 of their 60 eligible nurses accomplish certification for a rate of 20%. These combined totals allowed cardiac services to increase its overall certification percentage to 29%, the highest for any nursing division in our hospital.

DISCUSSION

We achieved much success with improving certification rates when we used tenets of employee engagement to guide our strategies. When nurses were fully engaged, they took responsibility for achieving certification. Certification was not mandated by leadership, and each nurse had a choice of whether to pursue it.

When the concept of certification was transformed from a burdensome task with little practical impact, to a meaningful validation of everyday work, nurses thought of certification differently. Nursing leaders were a key factor to our success. They imparted the shared vision that assisted in changing the perception of certification. They kept the certification initiative focused on employee engagement and not individual or unit competition. Allowing early adopters of the initiative to assist in creating the strategies ensured that these informal staff leaders were fully engaged from the onset.

Not every strategy was used by every department. In the telemetry units, the most effective strategy was staff-led study sessions. In lieu of study sessions, the critical care areas held case study discussion groups. Both strategies were safe venues for learning because everyone truly wanted to understand the material. Participants were invested not only in their own learning, but also their coworkers' learning. This encouraged a collegial sharing of knowledge for a shared purpose not always found in nursing. The engagement was tangible, as these groups created a sense of team.

The career opportunities and recognition associated with certification cannot be overlooked. These accomplishments are aligned with both the rational and emotional dimensions of engagement because they provide financial and career rewards, as well as a personal sense of achievement. The cardiac nurses have demonstrated important individual successes. They have been very involved with hospital shared governance and other committees, and more cardiac nurses have successfully achieved career ladder promotion in the past year than any other service line.

Certainly, not every eligible cardiac nurse has achieved certification. However, the culture shift has reached a critical mass. Nurses who were not part of the certification initiative are coming forward and wanting to know how to get certified. To date, 35 nurses have inquired about the next round of study groups. As more nurses are successful, their colleagues want to be a part of the certification experience. This emerging engagement from the previously unengaged is evidence of the paradigm shift within cardiac services.

Certification is now part of what we do in cardiac services. Our leaders continue to promote it and nurses understand that achieving certification is part of belonging to this specialty division. The individual benefits are identified, but the greater good for cardiac outcomes is the shared vision. Our patients deserve knowledgeable nurses committed to ongoing professional development, as evidenced through the certification and recertification processes. Magnet statistics aside, we will continue to promote certification as the right thing to do.

REFERENCES

1. American Nurses Credentialing Center. Magnet recognition program application manual. Silver Spring (MD): Author; 2008.
2. Simolenski M. Eight great reasons supporting nurse certification. Ohio Nurses Rev 2009;84(4):1–5.
3. Cary A. Data driven policy: the case for certification research. Policy Polit Nurs Pract 2000;1(3):165–71.
4. Kendall-Gallagher D, Blegen MA. Competence and certification of registered nurses and safety of patients in intensive care units. Am J Crit Care 2009; 18(2):106–14.
5. Fitzpatrick JJ, Campo TM, Graham G, et al. Certification, empowerment, and intent to leave current position and the profession among critical care nurses. Am J Crit Care 2010;19:218–26.
6. Craven H. Recognizing excellence: unit-based activities to support specialty nursing certification. Medsurg Nurs 2007;16(6):367–72.
7. American Association of Critical Care Nurses certification survey. AACN Web site. Available at: http://www.aacn.org/wd/certifications/content/benefitsofcertwhitepaper.pcms?menu=certification. Accessed August 18, 2010.
8. Byrne M, Valentine W, Carter S. The value of certification—a research journey. AORN J 2004;79(4):825–35.
9. Seijts GH, Crim D. What engages employees the most or, the ten C's of employee engagement. Available at: http://www.iveybusinessjournal.com/article.asp?intArticle_ID=616. Accessed September 1, 2010.
10. Rutledge T. Getting engaged: thse new workplace loyalty. Toronto (ON): Mattanie Press; 2005.
11. Melcrum Research. Employee engagement: how to build a high-performance workforce. Washington, DC: Melcrum Publishing; 2005.

12. Baumruk R. The missing link: the role of employee engagement in business success. Workspan 2004;47:48–52.
13. Richman A. Everyone wants an engaged workforce: how can you create it? Workspan 2006;49:36–9.
14. Shaw K. An engagement strategy process for communicators. J Comm Manag 2005;9(3):26–9.
15. Manion J. Inspired staff can see through hard times. Hosp Health Netw 2009; 83(3):10.
16. Maslach C, Schaufelli WB, Leiter MP. Job burnout. Annu Rev Psychol 2001;52: 397–422.

The Outcomes of Magnet Environments and Nursing Staff Engagement: A Case Study

Valentina Gokenbach, RN, DM*, Karen Drenkard, PhD, RN, NEA-BC

KEYWORDS

- Nursing • Magnet designation • Magnet journey
- Nursing staff engagement

A group of bold nurse researchers used a unique approach to better understand the nursing shortage that was unfolding during the 1980s. High registered nurse (RN) turnover and vacancy rates were affecting most health care organizations during an era when increasing opportunities other than nursing were available for smart and capable young women. Yet a group of hospitals had low turnover and vacancy rates and had no trouble recruiting and retaining nurses. These researchers decided to study the issues that were right with the health care organizations, rather than investigate what was wrong. A study was commissioned by the American Academy of Nursing's (AAN) Task Force on Nursing Practice in Hospitals.[1] They identified 163 hospitals to identify and describe variables that created an environment that attracted and retained well-qualified nurses who promoted quality patient care. As a result of their study, there were a group of 41 hospitals that were described as "magnet" hospitals because of the characteristics they all shared, and through these elements they were able to attract and retain professional nurses. These characteristics became known as "Forces of Magnetism."

The American Nurses Association created the American Nurses Credentialing Center (ANCC) as a subsidiary in 1990. This subsidiary exists so that credentialing programs and services can be offered to nursing professionals. The Magnet Recognition Program for Excellence in Nursing Services was created in 1990 to offer an organizational credential for outstanding nursing care delivery.

The Magnet program is based on the research and evidence for nursing excellence in health care organizations. In 2007, the Commission on Magnet worked with

Magnet Recognition Program, American Nurses Credentialing Center, 8515 Georgia Avenue, Silver Spring, MD 20910, USA
* Corresponding author.
E-mail address: dr.val@comcast.net

Nurs Clin N Am 46 (2011) 89–105
doi:10.1016/j.cnur.2010.10.008
0029-6465/11/$ – see front matter © 2011 Published by Elsevier Inc.

researchers to introduce a new model. The model is based on Donabedian's[2] quality framework and includes structure, process, and outcome measures. There are 5 areas of the new Magnet model:

- Transformational leadership
- Structural empowerment
- Exemplary professional practice
- New knowledge, innovations, and improvements
- Empirical outcomes.

THE MAGNET MODEL

As stated, the new Magnet model uses Donabedian's[2] structure-process-outcome model as a unifying framework for quality (**Fig. 1**). Structure includes the organizational and physical characteristics of an organization that are foundational; processes are the ways in which work is accomplished, and the outcomes are the results of the structure and processes. The Magnet model has structural requirements, process requirements, and outcome requirements for each of the areas that are assessed for excellence. The requirements, known as sources of evidence, are based on evidence and are in the areas of transformational leadership; structural empowerment; exemplary professional practice; new knowledge, innovation, and improvements; and empirical outcomes. Outcomes evidence is required in multiple areas.

The Magnet credential is unique in that it requires health care organizations to demonstrate excellence in the following 3 areas: patient satisfaction, nurse satisfaction, and nurse-sensitive clinical outcome data. Each organization describes and demonstrates that they have superior performance in these realms, and data are presented during the review process. These indicators need to outperform the midpoint of a national benchmarking tool in use by the organization. This requirement raises the bar for Magnet organizations to be accountable to outcomes, as well as structure and process.

When an organization decides to embark on the Magnet journey, nursing leaders conduct an initial assessment of the standards and determine the areas of strength and organizational gaps from the requirements. Identification of areas for improvement and development of action plans should be reviewed before submitting an application. The application is first submitted and then approved with a timeline provided to

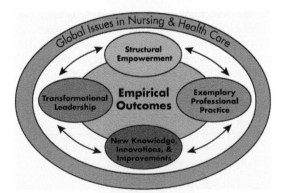

Fig. 1. The magnet model. (*Courtesy of* the American Nurses Credentialing Center, Silver Spring, MD. © 2008 American Nurses Credentialing Center. All rights reserved. Reproduced with the permission of the American Nurses Credentialing Center.)

the organization for subsequent submission of supporting documentation demonstrating compliance to the Magnet standards or "essentials." The applications and documents are peer reviewed and if the organization can demonstrate meeting the threshold of excellence, a site visit is scheduled. A site visit is conducted to clarify, amplify, and validate the findings from the written documentation. The site visit is a rigorous and comprehensive process and allows the organization to demonstrate the essential forces of magnetism in the organization.[3]

STATE OF THE CURRENT LITERATURE AND THE OUTCOMES IN MAGNET HOSPITALS

Research has been growing that shows a relationship between Magnet status and improved patient outcomes. Both quality outcomes and patient safety outcomes are linked to Magnet hospitals. Research comparing Magnet organizations with non-Magnet organizations have found Magnet recognition to be associated with lower rates of falls.[4] In one study,[4] fall rates were 10.3% lower in Magnet hospitals. In addition, decreased rates of pressure ulcers have been linked to Magnet status.[5–7] A study of hospitalized patients with hip fractures demonstrated that those Medicare beneficiaries hospitalized in Magnet hospitals were less likely to develop a decubitus ulcer (M.C. Rosenberg. Do Magnet recognized hospitals provide better care? Presented at the 2009 Magnet National Conference, Louisville, Kentucky, Unpublished data.). This was validated in a study by Goode and Blegen.[8]

Magnet characteristics have been linked to the patient safety climate. Highly qualified and satisfied staff nurses have a positive impact on patient safety as well as the prevention of adverse events that can harm patients. Findings from a study by Hughes and colleagues[9] demonstrated that nursing workgroups and managerial commitment to safety were the two most strongly positive attributes of the patient safety climate. Additional research shows that failure to retain nurses contributes to avoidable patient deaths.[10,11] In addition, hospitals with better educated nurses have lower mortality rates.[12]

Perhaps the strongest links have been demonstrated between Magnet hospital status and nurse satisfaction, which is a precursor to retention. There is a strong history of linkages between the structural components of Magnet hospitals, including autonomy in practice, structural empowerment, and participation in decision-making opportunities, and high levels of nurse and work satisfaction.[6,13–17] In turn, this positive work satisfaction results in lower vacancy and turnover rates, as validated by Lacey and colleagues'[18] research examining the impact on intent to stay. Magnet hospital nurses are more likely to stay than those who do not work in Magnet hospitals. This leads to cost savings for hospitals that may be struggling with high turnover and vacancy costs in an era of resource constraints.

Magnet organizations demonstrate excellent outcomes, especially related to workforce, and this is reflected in the low turnover of 9.9% and vacancy rate of 2.6% of Magnet hospitals across the United States.[19] There are reported national vacancy averages in 2007 at 8.1% to 16.0%, depending on the specialty and the region of the country.[20] In the past 12 months, part-time employees and RNs who may have been out of the workforce have been reported returning because of the economic recession. Nonetheless, as the economy improves, the nursing shortage will worsen, and organizations that have a compelling workplace environment will attract nurses.

STAFF ENGAGEMENT AND NURSE SATISFACTION

Engagement is defined as "being physically, mentally and emotionally connected to work."[21] Nurses who are engaged "feel a sense of ownership, loyalty, and dedication to create a safe environment for patients and an effective and efficient working environment. Engagement is a primary, critical component of patient safety and quality of care."[21,22] Methods to determine if nurses are engaged in their work often include surveys that measure variables that relate to the level of engagement. The Gallup organization completed a study of 200 hospitals and evaluated the relationship between nurse engagement and mortality and complication rates. Their results, including regression analysis, concluded that nurse engagement is the number one predictor of mortality variation across hospitals.[23] The results of the Gallup research also linked nurse engagement to quality care, including complications and mortality rate. They concluded that people and their level of engagement in work is the most important factor, especially related to nurses at the bedside.[23] The top 3 predictors of mortality, in order of significance, statistically significant at P less than .05, are the engagement level of nurses, the number of nurses/total patient day, and percentage of overtime hours per year.

Another study, completed by Mackoff and Triolo,[24] evaluates the impact of the level of engagement of nurse managers. In addition, they worked to identify the characteristics of engaged nurse managers. The researchers interviewed 30 nurse managers using the Nurse Manager Engagement Questionnaire (NMEQ) tool. The NMEQ, "shaped in an appreciative inquiry format, measures positive attributes and emphasizes experiences and long-term values in individuals and organizations that are associated with nurse manager engagement."[24–26] The study identified the characteristics of an engaged nurse leader and includes one who is mission driven, generatively (meaning developing others in the next generation), and ardor.

The question for nurse leaders then is how engaged and satisfied are the nurses are in their organization. Are the nurses loyal and committed to the organization and their jobs as nurses? Does the workplace environment have structures and processes in place for nurses so that they can impact patient care outcomes?

The Magnet criteria provide the roadmap for the structures and processes that are required to create a workplace environment where nurses can thrive. An example of a hospital system where the Magnet model is fully enculturated is William Beaumont in Michigan. Their story is one of a journey that was traveled to ensure that nurses are fully engaged and that patient outcomes are at the highest level possible.

IMPLEMENTATION OF AN EFFECTIVE MAGNET ENVIRONMENT: A CASE STUDY

The organization under study is William Beaumont Hospital, a large, 1063-bed academic hospital and referral center in Southeast Michigan with close to 60,000 admissions. The organization is the only level one trauma center in Oakland County with 120,000 emergency visits annually. Other services include a children's hospital, oncology and radiation oncology, stroke certification, neurology and neurosurgery, bariatrics, orthopaedics, palliative and hospice care, transplant services, geriatrics, and full-service cardiac care inclusive of a large cardiac surgery program. The surgical department was recognized as one of the busiest in the country with close to 50,000 surgical cases a year. The hospital has had multiple specialties recognized in the US News and World Report,[27] and in 2009 *Nursing Professional Magazine*[28] recognized Beaumont as one of the top 100 hospitals for nurses to work.

The Beaumont health care system is the largest employer in Oakland County, with 14,000 full-time equivalent employees and $2.1 billion in revenue annually. The nursing organization of the Royal Oak division is large and complex with 3500 nursing staff on 32 inpatient nursing units varying in size from 20 to 118 beds. The services are divided into surgical services, medical services, maternal child health, and specialty services under separate nursing directors. Other nursing departments include Care Management, the Access Center, Nursing Resource Team, Rapid Response Team, and Trauma Services. All nurses that interface with the patients at the bedside report directly to the Chief Nursing Officer (CNO), and all other nurses in the organization have a dotted line relationship to the CNO. In support of nursing, other departments that collaborate with nursing such as Respiratory Therapy also report to the CNO.

BUILDING A CASE FOR MAGNET

Large, complex health care organizations pose great challenges with regard to communication, coordination, and engagement of staff for many reasons. Such was the case in this organization. Limited management resources and large units create communication challenges for not only the dissemination of vital information but also for the creation and maintenance of relationships whereby the nurses feel valued and appreciated by their leaders. A positive working relationship and feelings of being valued have been recognized as key drivers to the retention of staff in the workplace despite the industry.[29] Retention rates and turnover statistics historically were about 12% before beginning the Magnet journey. Vacancy rates hovered around an average of 4% and overtime rates were at 9%. To fill the vacancies created by the turnover and vacancies, overtime and premium pay were offered with the costs of premium pay reaching an all-time high of $1.8 million.

At the same time, changes in the local economy, coupled with intense competition of new local hospitals, created a threat of potential loss of nursing staff while financial constraints in the organization led to several rounds of staff reduction and reorganization. Some of these changes affected the nursing organization through the loss of leadership positions and the reduction of support staff, leaving a feeling of unrest among the nursing community. There was a sense that nursing morale during these challenging times was beginning to erode, which could lead to higher turnover rates and subsequently higher vacancy rates. The Essentials of Magnet survey was used as a tool to assess the work environment and readiness of the organization to successfully begin the Magnet journey and successfully achieve Magnet accreditation. The survey showed opportunities in several areas, including image and status of nurses in the organization, empowered work environment, physician-nurse relationships, nursing education, and research and leadership development. It was the goal of the CNO and the nursing leadership to create a positive and meaningful interface with the nursing staff, despite the challenges of size and complexity, and to begin the Magnet journey.

CREATING THE MAGNET STRUCTURE

Beginning the journey to Magnet seemed like a monumental task, and with an organization as large as Beaumont it was evident that there needed to be a comprehensive strategic plan and formalized structure to be successful (**Fig. 2**). With regard to the organization of the documents, survey process, and collection of evidence, nursing directors were aligned with a Magnet force that coincided with their area of interest and competence. The directors were accountable to work with the Magnet coordinator to complete the work and achieve aggressive deadlines.

In support of the director group, a very large Magnet team was assembled, composed of nurse representatives from every area of the organization to help maintain energy, build excitement, and inculcate the Magnet culture in their individual nursing areas. It was believed that although the Professional Nurse Council (PNC) would be intimately involved in the Magnet process as well, they needed to continue

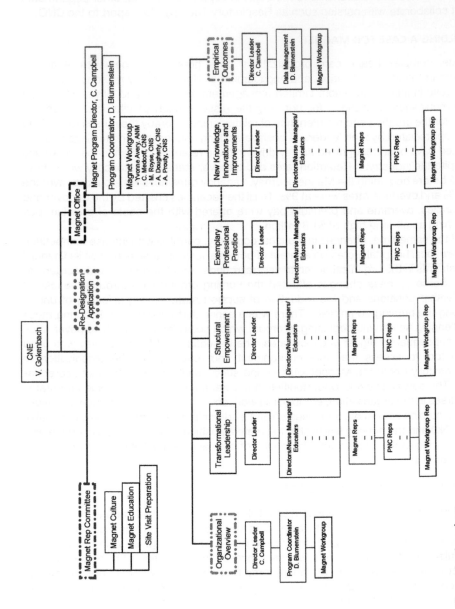

Fig. 2. Magnet organization chart.

their council work. With the size of the units and the number of nurses across the organization, it was decided that more manpower would be needed for coordination and communication. The Magnet team was expected to attend a 4-hour monthly meeting dedicated solely to the efforts of the Magnet journey and to align closely with their PNC representative and nurse leader. Magnet team members were also aligned under directors in the different areas of focus.

It was also the desire of the Magnet team to completely control the survey process and to be liaisons for the Magnet survey team. It was truly exciting to watch the creativity of the group as they developed trip-ticlike documents and who's who publications to help the surveyors understand the organization and the degree of complexity.

The Magnet team has now become part of the culture and the cornerstone of the survey process. Their work never ends and they work tirelessly to collect Magnet stories and maintain the energy on the various work units while working toward the next re-accreditation process.

IMAGE OF NURSING IN THE ORGANIZATION

Although the nursing organization was perceived by administration and the physician community as effective and safe, nursing lacked stature in the organization and was deemed subservient to the physicians and administration rather than viewed as partners in care. This was felt by the nursing staff on many levels including the marketing program for the hospital that focused only on the value of the doctors. It was important to assess the reasons for these perceptions and to create a framework whereby nurses would be viewed as valuable in the organization in a visible and meaningful way. Initially, the chief medical officer (CMO) of the organization at the time of the first survey was not in support of Magnet and found no value in the pursuit. He also felt that the money needed for accreditation would be better spent in other ways. Conversely, however, the hospital director at the time did support the desire to achieve Magnet and made the ultimate decision with the CNO to move forward. It was not until after the first accreditation that the CMO recognized the value of the Magnet brand when he attended a national CMO conference and the other CMO attendees were asking about Magnet and boasting that their organizations had achieved this prestigious designation. The CMO acknowledged at that time that he now appreciated the vision of the nursing organization to move forward in this direction.

CREATION OF A NEW NURSING MODEL

A high priority in enhancing the image of nursing began with the creation of a unique, comprehensive nursing model that supported the tenets of the Magnet environment and clearly mirrored the goals of the nursing organization and the espoused values. This model was termed the "Beaumont Nurse" and was created in collaboration with all nursing organizations in the corporation within the Professional Nurse Councils and with a delegate of nursing leadership (**Fig. 3**). The outer circle of the model included knowledge, communication, critical thinking, and philosophy of nursing as the foundation with further delineation of these categories in the inner circles. A massive and formal communication plan was developed to begin to introduce nursing staff to the model and to begin to inculcate these tenets into the culture. The "Beaumont Nurse" model now appears on every piece of nursing letterhead, on all policies and procedures, in all marketing materials, on the Web site, and also all minutes of committees and staff presentations.

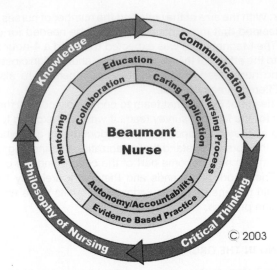

Fig. 3. Beaumont nurse model. (© 2003 William Beaumont Hospital. Used with Permission. All rights reserved. No part of this publication may be reproduced or transmitted in any form or by any means, electronic or mechanical, including photocopying, recording, or any information storage and retrieval system, without prior written permission.)

REDESIGN OF NURSING EDUCATION

Another strategy for improving the image of the nursing organization was the reengineering and redefining of the Nursing Development Department, which housed nursing educators and clinical nurse specialists. This department focused only on education with little attention on evidence-based practice, quality, or research. The new department was named the Division of Nursing Scholarship, Quality, and Research, which provided a broader scope highlighting the breadth and scope of nursing. This would also become the department that would coordinate the Magnet journey. Under a new director, creative new ideas and positions arose to provide a greater expansion of educational opportunities for the bedside nurse. One such position was called education specialists. Nurses interested in expanding their education experiences were selected from the units to provide in-services, help with orientation, and provide skills validation. In tandem with the education specialist position was the creation of a collaborative program with Oakland University to provide a comprehensive academic program for preceptor training. The creation of a robust clinical ladder program further stimulated interest on the part of the staff nurses to become more involved in the educational processes for nursing.

PROFESSIONAL IMAGE

Another initiative that proved to be valuable to the identity of the nursing organization was the selection of scrub colors that would clearly delineate nursing in contrast to the other disciplines. Nurses were able to select the color through a vote process and to rewrite the dress code policy. Ceil blue scrubs and white jackets were selected for all nurses throughout the organization. Pediatric and maternal child nurses would also wear the ceil blue but could wear a colorful jacket appropriate to help minimize stress in the pediatric population. No other department was allowed to pick ceil blue as their color choice. Other members of the nursing organization such as unit secretaries and nurse assistants chose colors as well. All published documents used for patient information included the nursing dress code for easy identification of the nursing staff.

RESEARCH

Before the beginning of the Magnet journey, the nursing organization lacked a strategy for an evidence-based approach and formal research. The reorganization of the Nursing Development department was important for the coordination of this goal and to provide leadership that would support nursing research and evidence-based practice at the bedside. Several off-site conferences were held for staff nurses to begin to demystify the concepts of research and increase confidence in the staff that they could become involved and be successful. Through the conferences, the attendees were expected to identify an area of research, process improvement, or evidence-based analysis and to create a change on their unit that was founded on the evidence. Mentors were assigned to support the staff through this journey with many wonderful projects identified and implemented. Several of the staff had their projects published in peer-reviewed journals, whereby other nurses had the opportunity to present their projects at national conferences as well as local university and hospital research events. It was also expected that all units would develop one evidence-based change project that was to be presented in a poster format annually during Nurse's Week. These were judged by nursing leaders and educators, staff, and physicians with awards and checks provided to the winners.

A greater level of support for research came from collaboration with Wayne State University through a contractual program to help with the education, designing, and conducting of nursing research projects. This was led through the creation of a collaborative committee that met monthly. This group was instrumental in the enhancement of the quality of nursing research in the organization.

The increased visibility of nursing research and scholarship helped to further improve the nursing image in the organization, especially with the physician group. Nurses became involved in many collaborative research projects and now are jointly presenting their research with physicians and other clinical colleagues. Nursing is also now well respected in the organization's research institute.

EMPOWERED NURSING WORKFORCE AND IMPROVED STAFF ENGAGEMENT

Kanter,[30] a proponent of empowerment, believed that organizations that allowed staff to make significant decisions of a substantive nature that affected their work environment had employees who were more engaged.[31] Several research studies suggest that feelings of empowerment also lead to employee engagement that leads to the intent of staff to remain in their jobs.[32] Kanter defined empowerment as the ability to make changes in the work environment through the mobilization of resources targeted to achieve the desired changes. This increased level of engagement was believed to lead to the improvement of organizational outcomes.[31] A formalized structure for empowerment was developed and implemented in 2002. This group was called the Professional Nurse Council (PNC); however, after a couple years of evolution it was decided that the structure of the group did not seem to support optimal performance and accomplishment of significant goals. An entire new model was designed and implemented that proved successful.

The original design of the PNC was based off the councilor model identified in the works of Timothy Porter-O'Grady, DM, EdD, APRN, FAAN. Four councils were in place including operations, policy and procedure, quality care, and research. The primary interest for accomplishing work was in the area of operations with less interest in the other councils. Individuals who were assigned to councils that they had little interest in lacked the drive and enthusiasm to produce significant outcomes. There needed to be a structure that capitalized on the interests and strengths of all members of the PNC.

The new council was based on a task-force model under the major tenets of operational design, nursing quality of care, evidence-based practice, and research. Seventy-two nurses representing all areas in the organization that employed nurses were elected by their peers and began meeting on a monthly basis for 8 hours to identify and deal with issues deemed important to the nursing staff. Each member was also given another 4 hours per month to work on projects as necessary. Members would be expected to commit to a 2-year term with 50% of the Council turning over on a yearly basis. It was believed that this would allow for new thinking with new membership while preserving experience with the remaining members of the group. Four domains of the council were established including hospital operations, education and research, policy and procedure, and quality. Issues within these 4 domains were addressed using a task force methodology.[33]

A chair and vice chair were elected by the members to organize and lead the functions of the PNC and to provide a linkage to nursing and hospital administration. Two nonvoting nurse managers and 1 nursing director were elected by the council to provide advice and help with implementation of programs and processes and to help secure funding when necessary. The elected leadership members would serve in that capacity for 1 year. The members of the PNC were expected to conduct unit-based council meetings and to work collaboratively with their respective managers to improve processes on their individual units.

It was also decided that this council would prove as a vehicle for the cultivation of new managers. A matriculated leadership program was developed to provide a comprehensive review of leadership topics, such as leadership theory, organizational theory, communications, health care economics, delegation, and emotional intelligence. This program also provided continuing education credits, increasing value to the members. To date, many open management positions are filled by current or past PNC members.

Along with the change to the task force model, a peer review component was also included for a portion of the monthly meeting. During the peer review segment of the meeting, best practices as well as areas of needed improvement were discussed in a case review format. These reviews also led to the identification of opportunities for work of the PNC.

The PNC has evolved over the years to become very well respected in the organization and a vital source of information to leadership before decision making at all levels. Every month, the council spends dedicated time with the CNO, the hospital director, and the CMO and is encouraged to openly share thoughts and feelings.

QUALITY OF CARE

The nursing organization has performed well through Joint Commission and other regulatory surveys and remained below benchmark for key nursing care and safety indicators, however lacked a visionary and cutting edge approach to nursing practice. Care of the patient was viewed primarily as physician driven without significant acknowledgment of the value of nursing in the delivery of care process. There was also a lack of recognition in the nursing community for contribution to the body of nursing research and information because of the lack of communicating accomplishments achieved in the organization.

Nursing was also not consistently represented in some important quality or process committees. A concerted effort was made to identify all committees engaged in quality and process issues and to add nursing staff as representatives to actively work on various projects collaboratively with the physicians. This provided visibility of the expertise of nursing leadership and highlighted the value of nursing input into these groups. This also allowed for the collapse of several committees that were meeting separately to now join together early in the process improvement effort.

To increase the sensitivity of the staff to the importance of nursing in the provision of care and as a component of the Magnet journey, the organization subscribed to the National Database for Nursing Quality Indicators (NDNQI). Data on nursing-sensitive indicators is now measured, benchmarked, and shared with the staff in a comprehensive and meaningful way. This led to the creation of several initiatives to improve the data especially in the area of falls, restraints, and pressure ulcers.

EFFECTIVE NURSING LEADERSHIP

The Essentials of Magnet survey also showed a need to improve the consistency of nursing leadership and to make a greater commitment to the growth of leaders in the organization. Nurses also felt that there were inconsistencies with communication and visibility of nursing leadership in the nursing areas.

COMMUNICATION

To develop consistency in communication, a program called "Talk to me" was created for all nursing leaders. This program not only highlighted the theories and strategies of fundamental communication but also set expectations for staff meetings, guidelines for feedback, and specific formats for meetings. Nursing leaders were also encouraged to attend formal communication programs offered through the hospital's development department and all leaders were expected to complete 40 continuing education credits in the area of leadership.

Nursing staff and leaders were brought together on a regular basis in various formats to provide information exchange and time of open sharing with nursing leaders. The Nurse Executive Leadership Forum (NELF) was held on a monthly basis and led by the CNO. In this meeting, all nursing leaders and clinical nurse specialists received key information about the organization from the CNO and developed action plans for issues related to nursing. A subset of the NELF was the Nursing Administrative Team composed of all nursing managers. The managers were empowered to address issues specific to their level of leadership and to handle issues that affected care at the bedside, thus moving decision making closer to the bedside.

Several forums for nursing staff were also created. A monthly focus group meeting called "Breakfast with Val" was initiated, whereby nurses were invited from all areas of the organization to have breakfast with the CNO and to discuss strategies to improve the nursing organization. Another monthly meeting was the Nursing Town Hall where all staff was invited to a very large forum in the auditorium to hear information and to share concerns, thoughts, rumors, and recommendations. Along with the meetings, a CNO blog was created to communicate to the staff and allow for comments and recommendations online.

The visibility of the nursing leadership team continued to be a concern. The CNO began to dedicate 4 hours a week to working a different unit and spending quality time with the nursing staff. Wearing scrubs and shadowing staff proved to be one of the best ways to begin to understand first hand, issues on the various units and to work with the staff to identify solutions and then garner support. Outcomes of these experiences have led to staffing changes, equipment purchases, changes in nursing support systems, and improvement of processes on the floors. These experiences have been transformational for both the CNO and the nursing staff. Nursing directors and mangers were also expected to wear scrubs and to work the units periodically as well. Board members and other senior leaders also took time to wear scrubs and shadow nurses, which helped demonstrate the challenges and enhance support of the nursing community at the corporate and board levels.

RELATIONSHIP WITH THE MEDICAL COMMUNITY

Improved relationships with the medical community continue to be a challenge. A change in leadership of the CMO helped to move this initiative forward to a new level, as the new medical leadership voiced an inherent value for nursing and personally had a willingness to become engaged. Other visible changes were made to help align nursing and medical leadership including moving the offices of the CNO and CMO next to each other to allow for easier access between leaders and improved communication.

Plans are under way to realign units and patient care departments to provide more consistent medical teams who can then become familiar and comfortable with the local nursing team, resulting in increased teamwork. The CNO also attends all of the medical executive meetings and other medical departmental meetings to provide a continual interface with nursing.

OUTCOMES

It is believed at Beaumont that the journey to Magnet and the structure that was developed provided a framework to dramatically improve the quality of the nursing organization. The financial return on investment of the Magnet journey is also irrefutable within our organization and evident in the outcomes from both patient and staff perspectives. The outcomes realized in the nursing departments contributed to improved communication and functionality of other departments within the organization as well.

Outcomes: Manpower Turnover and Vacancy Rates

Probably the most compelling evidence for the effect of a Magnet environment lies in the manpower statistics. Turnover rates fell over the time of the Magnet journey from 13% to 8% in 2009 with an anticipated turnover rate of 6% in 2010 (**Fig. 4**). A subsequent decrease in vacancy rate was realized from a high of 6% to 4% in 2009 and is projected to be at 3% for 2010. The Magnet designation also helped with recruitment of nurses to the hospital, which led to a waiting list of nurses wishing to be employed by the first and only Magnet hospital in Michigan.

Unscheduled sick calls decreased from 66,000 hours in 2003 to 56,000 in 2009 with about 56,000 projected for 2010 (**Fig. 5**). It was believed that this drop in unscheduled sick calls has been related to higher satisfaction within nursing, thus allowing the nurse managers to better predict staffing levels and help reduce the overtime usage, again supporting satisfaction.

Overtime percentages continue to drop since 2002 to an all-time low of 3% in 2009 with the same projection of 3% in 2010 (**Fig. 6**). An acute need to use overtime staffing led to the creation of premium pay to help incentivize staff to work more hours. Because of the decrease of the overtime hours, premium pay was eliminated in 2009 and has not been needed in 2010. The cost of the program was $8.1 million dollars for the 6 years of its use. The annual costs were as high as $1.8 million dollars alone in 2 of the 6 years.

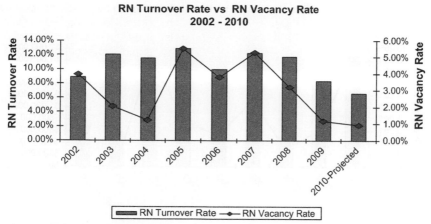

Fig. 4. Manpower and vacancy rates.

Outcomes: Manpower Staff Satisfaction

The Gallup measurement of staff engagement was instituted in 2007. The first measurement of the nursing staff showed a score of 3.75 on a 5.00 scale. This score improved in 2009 to 4.00 and slightly decreased in the beginning of 2010 to 3.96 (**Fig. 7**). Further analysis suggested that in 2010, the staff felt less appreciated by the organization because of pay cuts, a wage freeze for 2 years, and loss of 1 week of combined time off. The organization continues to struggle with the economic downturn, which has resulted in continued concerns on behalf of the staff with regard to their financial future and job security. The scores of the Essentials of Magnet survey continued to improve over time in all areas of study.

Outcomes: Patient Satisfaction

Several studies on the link between an empowered, engaged workforce and patient satisfaction have suggested that responses to the work environment are reflected in the patient satisfaction scores.[31] Press Ganey scores for inpatient nursing fell far below the goals set by the organization in the years before Magnet designation.

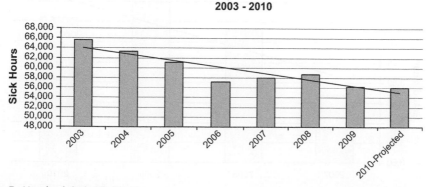

Fig. 5. Unscheduled sick hours.

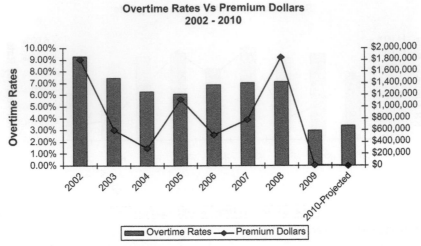

Fig. 6. Overtime and premium pay.

Following the beginning of the Magnet journey, scores have continued to improve (**Fig. 8**). It was decided to use a control chart methodology to identify special cause variation in the progress of the outcomes. In August of 2006, the hospital was under construction, which is believed the special cause for the short period of lower scores. The emergency center also showed a nice improvement in patient satisfaction scores over time with positive special cause variation in later years. All programs to improve the patient experience were designed, implemented, and augmented by the nursing staff.

Outcomes: Nurse-Physician Relationships

Analysis and improvement of the nurse-physician relationships began with the use of the Essentials of Magnet survey. In 2004, only 39% of the nursing staff felt that there

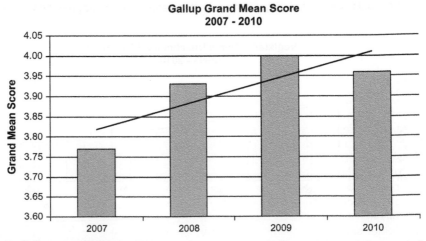

Fig. 7. Gallup engagement scores.

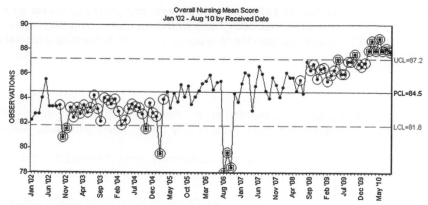

Fig. 8. Inpatient Press Ganey control chart.

were good relationships between nurses and the medical staff. In 2006, the score improved to 61.2%. Beginning in 2007, the NDNQI survey was used and also showed improvement from 2.85 on a 5.00 scale in 2007, 2.98 in 2008, and 2.96 in 2009. Efforts to improve the relationship continue. Subjectively, there is a general feeling that the physicians have a greater level of respect for the nursing team, which is reflected in the perception of improved relationships.

Outcomes: Quality Indicators

One of the greatest advantages of the Magnet journey was the focus on an evidence-based approach and the use of research for process improvements. Before this shift in focus, the organization was insulated in their approach to change, and attempted improvements in processes resulted in limited and often unsustainable success initiatives. In retrospect, this insulated approach truly limited creativity and hindered progress and true change. The focus on an evidence-based approach has enlightened the nursing team and leaders to new, scientific, best practices, both within and outside the system. With new programs and process change, there is now the discipline to effectively evaluate results using appropriate metrics and to change course when indicated. It is believed that this approach led to several strategies that improved nursing outcomes in the areas of falls, pressure ulcers, and restraints. Although not quantified for the purpose of this article, improvement of nursing quality has translated to the reduction of resources and a decrease in complication rates along with a subsequent decrease in length of stay at our organization.

SUMMARY

To ensure that nursing as a profession is recognized for the value we provide to our organizations, communities, and the world, a consistent level of practice and professionalism will be necessary. Consistency across the profession can be achieved through support of the framework and structures required for the process of attaining Magnet designation. This article is a case study of an organization that on all levels from economic, manpower, quality, and safety has benefited from the Magnet journey. Following the accreditation of Beaumont Royal Oak, the Beaumont Troy hospital successfully achieved Magnet with the goal of Magnet designation at the Beaumont Grosse Pointe site in the future, thus setting the bar high within our system. The Magnet journey has allowed the nursing staff to feel proud of the work they do, feel empowered and in control of their work environment, and ultimately valued by the organization. The commitment has been made by this transformed nursing organization to continually strive to maintain the "magnetized" culture supporting a pursuit of excellence.

REFERENCES

1. McClure M, Poulin M, Sovie M, et al. Magnet hospitals: attraction and retention of professional nurses. Kansas City (MO): American Nurses Association; 1983.
2. Donabedian A. Explorations in quality assessment and monitoring: the definition of quality and approaches to its assessment. Ann Arbor (MI): Health Administration Press; 1980.
3. Application manual, Magnet Recognition Program. Silver Spring (MD): American Nurses Credentialing Center; 2008.
4. Dunton N, Gajewski B, Taunton RL, et al. Nursing staffing and patient falls in acute care hospital units. Nurs Outlook 2004;52(1):53–9.
5. Gardner JK, Fogg L, Thomas-Hawkins C, et al. The relationships between nurses' perceptions of the hemodialysis work environment and nurse turnover, patient satisfaction, and hospitalizations. Nephrol Nurs J 2007;34(3):271–81.
6. Laschinger HKS, Fingan JE, Shamian J, et al. A longitudinal analysis of the impact of workplace empowerment on work satisfaction. J Organ Behav 2004; 25:527–45.
7. Waldman JD, Kelly F, Arora S, et al. The shocking cost of turnover in healthcare. Health Care Manage Rev 2004;29(1):2–7.
8. Goode C, Blegen M. The link between nurse staffing and patient outcomes. National Magnet Conference abstract and presentation at 2009 Magnet conference 2009. Louisville (KY).
9. Hughes L, Chang Y, Mark B. Quality and strength of patient safety climate on medical surgical units. Health Care Manage Rev 2009;34(1):19–28.
10. Aiken LH, Smith HL, Lake ET. Lower Medicare mortality rates among a set of hospitals known for good nursing care. Med Care 1994;32(8):771–87.
11. Aiken LH, Sochalski J, Lake ET. Studying outcomes of organizational change in health services. Med Care 1997;35(Suppl):NS6–N18.
12. Aiken LH, Clarke SP, Cheung RB, et al. Education levels of hospital nurses and patient mortality. JAMA 2003;290(12):1–8.
13. Smith H, Tallman R, Kelley K. Magnet hospital characteristics and northern Canadian nurses' job satisfaction. Can J Nurs Leadersh 2006;19(3):73–86.
14. Rondeau KV, Wagar TH. Nurse and resident satisfaction in magnet long-term care organizations: do high involvement approaches matter? J Nurs Manag 2006;14(3):244–50.
15. Schmalengerg C, Kramer M. Essentials of a productive nurse work environment. Nurs Res 2008;57(1):2–13.
16. Ulrich BT, Buerhaus PI, Donelan K, et al. Magnet status and RN views of the work environment and nursing as a career. J Nurs Adm 2007;37(5):212–20.
17. Laschinger H, Shamian J, Thomson D. Impact of magnet hospital characteristics on nurses' perceptions of trust, burnout, quality of care, and work satisfaction. Nurs Econ 2001;19(5):209–19.
18. Lacey SR, Cox KS, Lorfing KC, et al. Nursing support, workload, and intent to stay in Magnet, Magnet aspiring and non-Magnet hospitals. J Nurs Adm 2007; 37(4):199–205.

19. Magnet characteristics on American Nurses Credentialing Center. Web site. Available at: http://nursecredentialing.org/Magnet/ProgramOverview/Magnet-Characteristics.aspx. Accessed August 23, 2010.
20. The 2007 State of America's Hospitals – taking the pulse. Chicago (IL): American Hospital Association publication; 2007.
21. Tim T. Evidence based strategies to address nurse manager engagement. Okla Nurse 2009;54:19.
22. Simpson MR. Engagement at work: a review of the literature. Int J Nurs Stud 2009;46:1012–9.
23. Gallup Web site. Nurse engagement key to reducing medical errors. Available at: http://www.gallup.com/poll/20629/nurse-engagement-key-reducing-medical-errors. aspx. Accessed August 23, 2010.
24. Mackoff B, Triolo P. Why Do Nurse Managers Stay? Building a Model of Engagement: Part 1, Dimensions of Engagement. J Nurs Adm 2008;38(3):118–24.
25. Mackoff B, Triolo P. Why Do Nurse Managers Stay? Building a Model of Engagement: Part 2, Cultures of Engagement. J Nurs Adm 2008;38(4):166–71.
26. DiJon F. The culture of nursing engagement: a historical perspective. Nurs Adm Q 2010;34(1):18–29.
27. Available at: http://health.usnews.com/best-hospitals/rankings. Accessed December 1, 2010.
28. Available at: http://www.beaumonthospitals.com/awards-honors. Accessed December 1, 2010.
29. Nedd N. Perceptions of empowerment and intent to stay. Nurs Econ 2006;24(1): 13–8.
30. Kanter RM. Men and women of the corporation. 2nd edition. New York: Harper Collins Publishers, Inc; 1993.
31. Vahey DC, Aiken LH, Sloan DM, et al. Nurse burnout and patient satisfaction. Med Care 2004;42(2):II-57–66.
32. Laschinger H, Finnegan J. Empowering nurses for work engagement and health in hospital settings. J Nurs Adm 2005;35(10):439–49.
33. Gokenbach V. A new model for nursing empowerment. J Nurs Adm 2007;37(10): 440–3.

The Rural Pipeline: Building a Strong Nursing Workforce Through Academic and Service Partnerships

Maureen Fitzgerald Murray, MS, RN, NE-BC[a],*,
Jeanne-Marie Havener, PhD, APRN, CNS, FNP[b], Patricia S. Davis, RN[a],
Connie Jastremski, MS, MBA, APRN[a], Martha L. Twichell, MS, RN, CCRN[c]

KEYWORDS

• Rural • Nursing workforce • Academic/service partnership

Building and sustaining a strong nursing workforce is challenging for any health care organization. This is particularly true for organizations in rural settings. This article describes the academic and service partnerships and programs that have been created and continue to evolve to support a continuously flowing "pipeline" of nursing students, novice nurses, competent nurse preceptors, and expert nurses who practice and teach as clinical faculty in a rural region. Bassett Medical Center was redesignated as a Magnet Hospital in July 2008, following initial designation in 2004. The goals of recruiting and retaining experienced nurses; sustaining a strong, stable, and highly qualified nursing workforce; and providing a supportive environment with transitional career and role pathways for nurses prompted several innovative programs and partnerships for this rural hospital. These programs and partnerships link academia and service within our community and are integral to support an organizational goal of "growing and enriching our own nurses."

THE RURAL CONTEXT FOR NURSING RECRUITMENT AND RETENTION

Nurses promote health, reduce health risks, treat illnesses and injuries, and assist those who are recovering from an illness, injury, or life-developmental transition. As

Authors have nothing to disclose.
[a] Nursing Department, Bassett Medical Center, 1 Atwell Road, Cooperstown, NY 13326, USA
[b] Department of Nursing, Hartwick College, 1 Hartwick Drive, Oneonta, NY 13820, USA
[c] Human Resources Department, Bassett Medical Center, 1 Atwell Road, Cooperstown, NY 13326, USA
* Corresponding author.
E-mail address: Maureen.murray@bassett.org

Nurs Clin N Am 46 (2011) 107–121
doi:10.1016/j.cnur.2010.10.010
0029-6465/11/$ – see front matter © 2011 Elsevier Inc. All rights reserved.
nursing.theclinics.com

consumers of nursing services, patients, families, employers, third party payers, and society are negatively affected by nursing shortages and workforce instability.[1]

In 2005 the federal Bureau of Health Professions reported a shortage of 13,000 nurses in New York; this was projected to reach 37,000 by 2015.[2] Current nurse shortages vary by geographic regions, but rural regions are faced with specific challenges, including reduced population density, out-migration of skilled workers, an aging workforce, and an increase in the aging patient population.[3] Bassett Healthcare Network (**Box 1**) is a vertically integrated enterprise serving an 8-county, rural upstate New York population in an area the size of the state of Connecticut. Several counties in this region are classified as medically underserved or "Health Professionals Shortage Areas".[4]

There are many challenges inherent in advancing the educational preparation of working adults and particularly those in rural areas. These challenges include time to work and study while maintaining gainful employment and benefits, money to pay for courses and travel, geographic access to programs of study, competing work-life demands, the lack of successful role models, and the lack of incentives to pursue additional education.[5,6] Uniquely, advancement in the educational levels of the nursing workforce should be viewed as part of a sound local development initiative benefiting not only the local economy of the communities but also the population of the citizens in rural communities. A better-educated nursing workforce has been shown to improve patient outcomes as well as add to the pool of available human

---

Box 1
Overview of Bassett Healthcare Network

Nonprofit healthcare network servicing patients in a 8-county area (approximately 7000 sq miles) of rural central New York

Bassett Medical Center is a 180-bed inpatient teaching facility and large ambulatory care clinic in the rural village of Cooperstown, New York

Affiliated with 4 smaller hospitals (2 of which are critical access hospitals with <50 beds) within a 50-mile radius

Two urgent care centers in small towns 35 and 45 miles away

Twenty-five health centers spread throughout the region

Nineteen school-based health centers

Services include trauma care (level II), comprehensive cancer care, heart institute, dialysis, and most medical and surgical specialties

Research institute conducts programs in basic and clinical sciences and population and public health studies

Closed-group medical practice with physicians and advanced practice nurses employed by the institution

Affiliation with Columbia University College of Physicians and Surgeons (in 2009, Bassett became a medical school campus of Columbia University *College of Physicians and Surgeons*)

Affiliation with Columbia-Presbyterian Medical Center in New York City

A total of 3200 employees

A total of 599 registered nurses (RNs) in hospital, ambulatory clinics, region

Magnet recognition by the American Nurses Credentialing Center (ANCC) since 2004

Data from Bassett Healthcare Network, Cooperstown, NY

capital, which in turn encourages greater innovation and the recruitment and retention of quality talent thus increasing the pool of nursing talent.[5,7,8]

According to sources, educational levels of adults in many rural counties remain far below the national average. Among other variables, fewer high-skill jobs and the lower likelihood of college attendance among rural youth account for this difference.[5,6] This is true in this rural region of New York, where only 17% to 22% of persons 25 years or older have earned a bachelor's degree.[9]

Given this, it is not surprising that nurses in this region are generally less well educated than nurses throughout the state and the nation. Two-thirds of New York State respondents to the National Sample Survey in 2004 indicated that they were diploma (33%) or associate degree (AD) prepared (35%); these values compared with 23% and 31%, respectively, in the national sample.[10] In the central New York region, of the more than 4000 RNs employed, nearly 80% are AD or diploma prepared, this value compares unfavorably to a statewide figure of 57.2%.[11]

Respondents to the 2008 Healthcare Association of New York State (HANYS) statewide survey[11] reported that RNs are the most challenging health care professionals to recruit and retain, a phenomenon more pervasive in rural areas. Owing to the differences in pay, benefits, career opportunities, and lifestyle factors, rural health care organizations have greater difficulty attracting and retaining nurses, particularly young nurses.[3,12] Although the current economic recession has created a temporary reprieve from the nursing shortage and exodus from the profession and jobs, steps to avert a catastrophe that will undermine the quality of health care once the reprieve ends are needed.[13]

These contextual variables present barriers to Bassett's retention and recruitment efforts, particularly as the organization moves to expand the scope and quality of its acute care services and establish itself as a regional leader in the provision of tertiary and specialty care. Creative approaches to these looming issues are a leadership and organizational challenge.

THE RURAL CONTEXT FOR PATIENT CARE

Regionally, the population served by Bassett is older and poorer than the upstate or statewide average in New York, with higher rates of the underinsured and uninsured. Also, the area's morbidity and age-adjusted mortality rates for certain cancers, diabetes, and cardiovascular and respiratory diseases exceed the New York State (excluding New York City) rate; the higher rates of premature death from these diseases are of particular concern.[14–16] Bassett's case mix index of 1.65 (1.63 in 2009, 1.65 in 2008) indicates a high acuity of patients compared with a typical inpatient case mix of 1.00 and represents an increase over the 2007 case mix index of 1.52. The average length of stay for inpatients remains quite low, at 4.60 days in 2009, but has increased steadily as the population ages and the complexity of cases treated and procedures performed increases. The high acuity level reflected in the case mix statistic is attributable to both the level of services available at Bassett and the health care status and needs of the area's population. Distance and transportation prevent many patients from having access to services. The working poor are often neglected or overlooked by Medicaid assistance and have no access to health care, thus decreasing the health status of the population. These gaps result in a greater number of patients using the hospital as a primary care provider and using resources when they are more likely to be very ill, thus requiring more complex nursing care.[16]

These 2 sets of circumstances, barriers to advancing education for rural nurses and communities of rural citizens with complex health needs and access issues, pose challenges. The following sections describe several programs that foster the recruitment and retention of nurses to Bassett. Seeking and nurturing partnerships with academic agencies provide synergy to this worthy work.

TUITION ASSISTANCE

For decades Bassett Healthcare has supported the pursuit of higher education for employees through tuition reimbursement. Guided by a tuition assistance policy that frames tuition assistance as a "promissory note," Bassett nurses have used the program to cover tuition fees at state university rates. After achieving a grade of C or higher, the nurse submits documentation for reimbursement. Previously, some local academic agencies had agreed to defer payment until the nurse was reimbursed, thus significantly reducing an economic burden for the employee, but this is no longer the case. The Tuition Assistance Program covers individual courses related to the nurse's practice or coursework within an educational program that confers a relevant degree. In 2009, tuition dollars spent toward advancing the education of nurses equaled $86,000.

THE PARTNERSHIP FOR NURSING OPPORTUNITIES PROGRAM

Bassett's nursing organization is committed to creating educational mobility pathways for nurses seeking to advance their skill and education while experiencing professional fulfillment.

The Partnership for Nursing Opportunities Program (PNOP) was conceived and implemented almost 10 years ago to remove some of the barriers to Bassett nurses advancing on the education pathway. This academic/service partnership model linked Bassett's CEO and President, and Bassett's Chief Nursing Officer with College Presidents and Nursing Chairs from 2 local colleges, the State University of New York in Delhi, New York, and Hartwick College in Oneonta, New York. Programs were collaboratively designed to attract Bassett nurses, as well as nonnurse employees, to participate in an affordable educational path to either an associate or a baccalaureate degree nursing education. Before this program, Bassett nurses wishing to advance their education would enroll and seek approval for tuition assistance but would have to individually negotiate a work schedule with the supervisor to allow time for classes and study.

The Partnership Program removes or eases the barriers to advancing education while allowing the student to remain employed. Bassett pays the tuition in full, and nurses commit to 1 year of full-time employment within the Bassett system for each year of tuition coverage. Required course schedules are offered in 2-day blocks and arranged in advance, allowing nurses to work a full- or part-time schedule in 3 workdays. From the beginning, the program designers built in time off that is not work or school related to promote healthy, balanced lifestyles and thus employee wellness and retention. Class days are known in advance, allowing automated scheduling systems to create schedules that incorporate the employed nursing student's unique scheduling needs without the need for individual negotiation. Such flexible work arrangements allow the student-employees to complete their course work with fewer scheduling conflicts. Some of the didactic and most of the clinical components of the curriculum are taught on the main Bassett campus for almost all semesters, thus eliminating excessive time and travel expenses for the students. The creation of academic cohorts allows students to benefit from a close-knit academic and social support network while discouraging attrition and encouraging collegiality. To provide additional support, a dedicated part-time Nursing Advisor to the Hartwick College

Partnership Program provides students with regular access to an academic advisor, and nearly half of a full-time Project Coordinator's position is devoted to coordinating the day-to-day operations of the program, recruiting candidates, and retaining enrolled nurses.

The model is similar to a work/study experience, as the students are hired as either *Licensed Practical Nurses (*LPNs) or RNs. The work component affords the students the ability to gain knowledge and experience while furthering their education and providing them with a salary and company benefits.

In 2002, the first LPN to RN cohort began the second year of the Associate Degree nursing (ADN) program at the State University of New York at Delhi; 8 years later, the success of this endeavor is evident in the results (**Table 1**). As the program has evolved, nonnurse employees have also taken advantage of the PNOP.

THE NEWEST PARTNERSHIP

As we looked for ways to continue to address our nursing, nurse faculty, and provider shortages, a program that offered a master's degree option was the next imperative. Working with the State University of New York Institute for Technology (SUNY IT) in Utica, New York, we built on elements of the original Partnership Program to establish a supported BS to MS track in 2008. For baccalaureate-prepared nurses electing to pursue graduate studies, 2 core courses are offered on the Bassett campus and are funded through the Tuition Assistance Program. At present, 6 students are enrolled. Enrolled students are preparing for advanced practice nursing roles in nursing practice, administration, or education. School projects are designed to address clinical,

Table 1
Partnership for nursing opportunities Bassett Medical Center

Delhi/ADN May 2003–May 2010		Hartwick College/BS September 2001–May 2010		Graduate School Partnership Program	
Bassett employed LPNs enrolled in the Bassett/Delhi Partnership Program	41	RNs from the Delhi Partnership who entered Hartwick College RN to BS Partnership Program	19	Hartwick College Partnership graduates currently in graduate school	22%
Newly recruited Graduate Practical Nurse candidates who enrolled in the Bassett/Delhi Partnership Program	46	RNs (not Delhi Partnership) who entered the Hartwick RN to BS Partnership Program	18		
Total employed graduate nurses who graduated from the Bassett/Delhi Partnership Program	87	Total employed RNs obtaining BS through the Bassett/Hartwick RN to BS Partnership Program	37		
Retention rate of Bassett/Delhi Partnership Program RNs (Retention is to date, includes 7 years of the program)	77%	Retention rate of BS RNs from the Bassett/ Hartwick Partnership Program	78%		

environmental, or scope-of-practice issues in the work setting, thus enriching the practice environment at Bassett.

Hartwick College recently launched an 18-month accelerated nursing program, the Rural Nursing Opportunities Program (RNOP), designed for local and regional residents with degrees in other areas who are interested in a career in nursing. Moving forward, the RNOP will bring senior nursing students to the Bassett campus to complete a 2-month clinical practicum that is integrated with a capstone socialization course and is the culmination of the program. Also, the program will create a curricular bridge with SUNY IT's RN to MS program such that graduates will earn 6 to 9 credits toward a master's degree.

The next step is to support an educational pathway to the doctoral level. The SUNY IT program has recently been approved to move forward with the development of a Doctor of Nursing Practice Program. Once started, it is planned to have nursing leaders at Bassett develop a partnership with that program as well.

BASSETT AS A CLINICAL SITE

Bassett is a clinical site for several local nursing schools. In addition to the Partnership Programs previously described, Bassett serves as the primary clinical site for student rotations in both the Hartwick College traditional 4-year bachelor of science in nursing program and the State University of New York (SUNY) at Delhi's 2-year associate of applied science in nursing program. In addition to traditional instructor-led student clinical groups, several precepted clinical practicum experiences are provided to students at Bassett from these and several other area colleges. Staff nurses serve as preceptors to these students who need to complete 40 to 128 hours of work at the bedside, thus adding to both the demands and potential rewards for nurse preceptors at the point of service. To encourage and reward those nurses who actively engage in the work of educating for the professions, the hospital's clinical ladder system, organized around the Magnet essentials, awards points toward credentialing or promotion for nurses serving as preceptors and faculty. Ongoing communication between academic faculty, nursing staff, and clinical leaders assures that nursing student experiences are optimal from the perspective of each organization. At the end of each semester, the nursing unit directors, hospital educators, and clinical faculty meet to evaluate the student experiences, clinical setting, relationships, and plans for future semesters. Expectations and clinical rotation schedules are discussed and planned. This group determines policies, procedures, and practices related to student rotations as needed.

BASSETT NURSES AS FACULTY

Many Bassett staff nurses also work as adjunct clinical faculty for area nursing schools. The close relationships and synergy engendered by the Partnership Programs afford an additional opportunity for skilled and seasoned staff nurses to evolve in their role while retaining the wealth of their talents at the point of service. Selected by the academic agencies, our own Bassett nurses can add "adjunct faculty" to their resumes. These nurses negotiate a semester-by-semester agreement with their work managers to reduce their work hours to allow time for faculty practice. The academic agencies compensate the nurses directly. In some cases, to accommodate the academic work schedule, the nurses cut down the number of hours worked at Bassett; however, becoming a part-time worker affects the availability and/or cost of employee benefits and has been dissatisfying to some.

As a potential response to this issue, Bassett partnered in August 2007 with Hartwick College and SUNY Delhi to implement a $250,000 grant from the Scriven Foundation (a charitable organization, founded in 1976 and focused on grants to health and medical agencies) to further strengthen and support the role of nursing adjunct clinical faculty. This grant funds additional adjunct faculty hours provided by expert Bassett nurses to supplement the on-site college faculty for selected clinical nursing groups. As a result, the nurses are able to maintain full-time employment with benefits at Bassett while enjoying the faculty role. In addition, the student to faculty ratios are decreased, allowing students to gain more experience in areas such as medication administration, performance of skilled procedures, and management of direct care for larger numbers of patients. Outcomes from this project include increased student, faculty, and staff satisfaction with the clinical experience and enhanced student preparation for future employment.

SUMMER NURSING INTERN PROGRAM

The Summer Nursing Intern program is another example of a successful service and academic partnership. Bassett has partnered with Hartwick College (and previously with Utica College) to serve as a clinical site for a highly competitive paid summer internship. Senior nursing students from several colleges apply for the opportunity to enroll in a 3-credit clinical course offered at the hospital. A faculty member from the college works closely with the students, preceptors, and hospital-based nurse educators to provide a 10-week clinical rotation, which includes a one-on-one relationship with a seasoned preceptor. The students develop a strong bond with their preceptors and gain the much desired real world clinical experience with patient assessments, care planning, medication administration, procedural skills, patient teaching, discharge planning, clinical problem solving, and documentation. Bassett pays tuition costs and wages (stipend) to the students. The students attend weekly seminars that include presentations by faculty and nurse experts from the hospital staff. Students end the semester with the formal presentation of an evidence-based change project on a quality or patient safety topic of their choice. This program serves as a "pipeline" for future recruitment to the hospital while contributing significantly to the academic experience of the students.

PROTECTING OUR NOVICE NURSES

Many new graduate nurses, particularly those from the ADN programs, with limited clinical placements, are not well prepared to deal with the demands of the acute care hospital environment. Without additional educational support, most new graduates experience difficulty in handling "the intense working environment, advanced medical technology and high patient acuity"; this has been noted to result in high rates of turnover among new graduate nurses.[17] Although Bassett recruits regionally and nationally, the constant shortage of graduating baccalaureate-prepared nurses who are willing and/or able to remain in or relocate to this rural region results in most new hires being drawn from the local, AD-prepared RN workforce.

To address this challenge to a stable, highly qualified nursing workforce, Bassett has developed a yearlong Nurse Residency for new graduates, which incorporates several academic resources into the program. The Nurse Residency program uses evidence-based intern and preceptor development strategies from programs such as the Vermont Nurses in Partnership Program[18] to improve the retention rates of new graduate nurses. In addition to improving nurse retention, the program aims to support the new graduate's transition to the workplace specifically through preparing the new graduate to handle the challenges of caring for groups of acutely ill patients with complex comorbidities and social situations.

The Nurse Residency program provides a combination of social support, didactic content, and skills training and validation as the new graduate makes the transition from student to practitioner. Using Benner's sentinel work, From Novice to Expert, as a theoretical framework,[19] the program promotes the smooth transition of the new graduate from the level of novice to advanced beginner or competent practitioner. In addition to a precepted 12-week orientation, new graduates in the program attend 8 weekly classes with a focus on case scenarios, simulation activities, skills validation, and critical problem solving. Additional full-day classes are spread throughout the first year to provide developmentally appropriate educational support. Nursing faculty from area colleges present classes or help mentor new graduates; simulation equipment is loaned from local nursing schools for use in this program.

A MAGNET ENVIRONMENT RETAINS NURSES

In early 2004, Bassett received the nation's highest recognition for nursing excellence, The Magnet Recognition Program, developed by the ANCC.

For a health care organization to be designated under the Magnet Recognition Program, it has to demonstrate Magnet "essentials," including transformational leadership, structures that empower nurses, exceptional nursing practices, and a culture that embraces new knowledge, innovations, and improvements. A magnet culture supports an evidence-based approach to care, empirically sound outcomes, and continuous improvements in the structures and processes of care; this cultural milieu has been shown to fulfill nurses' professional self views and satisfy and retain them in the work setting.[20]

Since the late 1980s, the Bassett nursing community has endorsed and embraced shared governance as a philosophy and structure by which decisions are made and through which professional excellence is achieved. The work of Dr Timothy Porter-O'Grady, DM, EdD, APRN, FAAN, shaped our organizational approach to shared governance. The 4 guiding principles of shared governance as identified by Dr Porter-O'Grady, partnership, equity, accountability, and ownership,[21] are used as a basis to guide our work together and support the recruitment and retention of nursing staff. The mission of the nursing community was rewritten in 2005 and emerged from focus group research with Bassett nursing staff at the point of service. Five years later, a team of nurses refreshing the nursing strategic plan found a "goodness of fit" with the Studer-based pillars,[22] which the organization had embraced as part of its overall plan, as well as the organization's mission, vision, and values (**Fig. 1**).

The Professional Practice Model, updated in advance of Bassett's 2008 Magnet Redesignation, describes the professional elements and shared decision-making groups that support the domain of professional nursing practice and that focus on the patient and family at the center (**Fig. 2**).

Education is so important at Bassett that it is listed as one of the 3 main components of the organization's mission. The organization has adopted a learning organization culture, based on the work of Peter Senge,[23] which is promoted by the Bassett Institute for Learning (BIL). The BIL is a multidisciplinary approach to fulfilling the educational mission of the organization by meeting the learning needs of Bassett staff and improving communication and access to these opportunities. The vision of the BIL is to "foster a culture that strives to have all of its members grow smarter and better." The BIL has a Web page that is accessible to employees from the Intranet with course

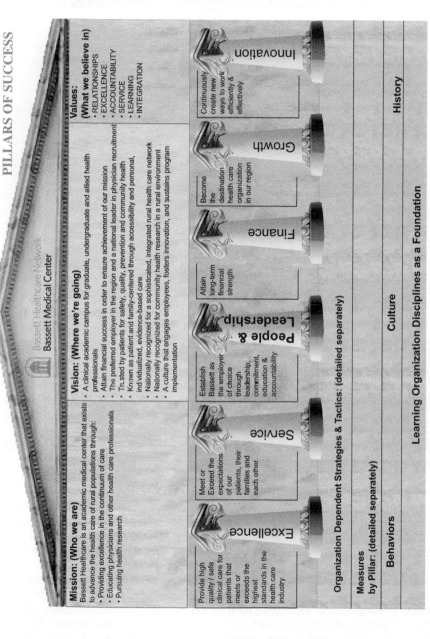

PILLARS OF SUCCESS

Bassett Healthcare Network
Bassett Medical Center

Mission: (Who we are)
Bassett Healthcare is an academic medical center that exists to advance the health care of rural populations through:
• Providing excellence in the continuum of care
• Educating physicians and other health care professionals
• Pursuing health research

Vision: (Where we're going)
• A clinical academic campus for graduate, undergraduate and allied health professionals
• Attain financial success in order to ensure achievement of our mission
• The preferred employer in the region and a national leader in physician recruitment
• Trusted by patients for safety, quality, prevention and community health
• Known as patient and family-centered through accessibility and personal, individualized, evidence-based care
• Nationally recognized for a sophisticated, integrated rural health care network
• Nationally recognized for community health research in a rural environment
• A culture that engages employees, fosters innovation, and sustains program implementation

Values:
(What we believe in)
• RELATIONSHIPS
• EXCELLENCE
• ACCOUNTABILITY
• SERVICE
• LEARNING
• INTEGRATION

Excellence
Provide high quality / safe clinical care for patients that meets or exceeds the highest standards in the health care industry

Service
Meet or Exceed the expectations of our patients, their families and each other

People & Leadership
Establish Bassett as the employer of choice through leadership, commitment, education & accountability

Finance
Attain long-term financial strength

Growth
Become the destination health care organization in our region

Innovation
Continuously create new ways to work efficiently & effectively

Organization Dependent Strategies & Tactics: (detailed separately)

Measures by Pillar: (detailed separately)

| Behaviors | Culture | History |

Learning Organization Disciplines as a Foundation

Fig. 1. Pillars of success. (*Courtesy of The Bassett Healthcare Network; with permission.*)

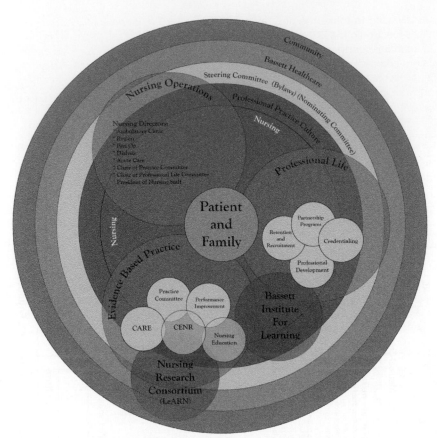

Fig. 2. Professional Practice Model for nursing staff at Bassett Medical Center. CARE, Council to Advance Research and Evidence-Based Nursing Practice; CENR, Center for Evidence Based Nursing and Research; LeARN, Leatherstocking Area Alliance for Research in Nursing.

listings, on-line course registration, on-line courses and learning modules, training videos, and a link to the HealthStream, Inc learning management system.

Abundant opportunities for ongoing educational and professional development, as well as a tradition of offering high-quality presentations on relevant nursing topics, bring and retain skillful nursing staff to Bassett's Magnet environment. Patient care is strengthened by a vital and comprehensive approach to life-long learning that is foundational to the BIL. As a provider unit for continuing education contact hours, Bassett offered in 2009 more than 50 continuing education programs that totaled 114 contact hours, with more than 1000 attendees.

Ten full-day continuing education conferences, which faculty and students often attend, are offered on-site at Bassett each year with high participation from staff nurses. Nursing Grand Rounds (NGR) is offered twice monthly. Both of these programs provide ANCC-approved continuing education hours for participants. At NGR, staff nurses, nurse leaders, community-based nurses, and faculty from local academic agencies, alone or in a team from a practice area, deliver hour-long case presentations and other evidence-based programs to illustrate the nursing process in action in the care of individuals, groups, and communities. Teleconferencing is routinely used to make the programs widely available to nurses and agencies in the region. Electronic messages to all Bassett nurses, affiliate hospitals, and community and academic partners announce the event, title, presenters, and learning objectives. Posters and overhead messages alert the on-site clinical faculty to attend along with their students. A close relationship between continuing education nurse planners and faculty brings the academicians as regular presenters. A quarterly mortality and morbidity focus has been inserted into the NGR schedule. Honoraria for outside speakers have been budgeted. Programs are recorded directly to a Polycom RSS 2000, a centralized server for recording, streaming, and archiving multimedia conferences. This allows for live streaming of presentations, with the option for later viewing at times more convenient to nursing staff and student groups who might not be able to leave the practice area or who work an off-shift.

Nursing Research Evening is an annual event scheduled on or near the birthday of Florence Nightingale, the first nurse scientist. More than 80 nurses attend the event, which showcases research and scholarly work from a variety of nursing professionals—student nurses, our own partnership students, nurses, administrators, and faculty from Bassett and the region. Our regional academic agencies often provide the keynote speaker for the event.

A Professional Nursing Pathway (Bassett's clinical ladder), based on Benner's model of skill acquisition in nursing[19] and overseen by the Credentialing Committee, links academia and service in yet another way. The Pathway was initially developed around the 14 Forces of Magnetism. A variety of professional activities and behaviors, demonstrated in a professional portfolio, are linked to the accumulation of points needed for promotion and for maintaining a certain level on the Pathway. Educational degrees obtained, academic credits earned during a semester, experience as faculty, written exemplars, and external presentations are some of the ways nurses can generate points in the program. The Pathway provides a "pull" culture as nurses assimilate professional practice activities and are pulled toward educational advancement.

REWARDS OF A PARTNERSHIP PROGRAM

The individual rewards of the partnering efforts described in this article are numerous. Those who have engaged in the PNOP have reaped the benefit of a high-quality educational experience at little cost (books, transportation, and the usual time and effort) while maintaining steady employment with a pay check and benefits package. Beyond this, however, is the transformative nature of the educational experience, one that opens new doors of opportunity to the graduates as professionals and as wage earners. But, in a larger sense, educational opportunities such as these allow students to view themselves and their place within the organization differently, that is, they feel recognized and rewarded for the contributions that they make. They also become more engaged as organizational and/or professional citizens. Indeed, many of the PNOP graduates continue to advance their education, take on leadership positions within the organization, join professional organizations, and take on the role of nurse preceptors or nursing faculty.

From an organizational perspective, implementation of the PNOP has afforded career mobility opportunities to nonlicensed employees, LPNs, and RNs within the system, thus, in theory, attracting talented employees to the organization, enhancing their job satisfaction, and retaining their skills as valued employees. As recruitment and retention tools, these programs have creatively addressed the regional nursing shortage and the shortage of a well-educated nursing workforce. Addressing nurse retention has positive economic benefits for the organization because every percentage point in the nurse turnover rate is said to represent about $300,000 annually, and hospitals that perform poorly relative to nurse retention spend, on average, about $3.6 million dollars more than those organizations that are top performers.[24] In addition, a more educated work force has added to the human and social capital available within the organization and region,[5] thus enhancing the professional culture

Annual Turnover RN/LPN and all Employees

Data from lawson BH219 Retention Rate report, through October 2009. Current Year represents current monthly turnover annualized.

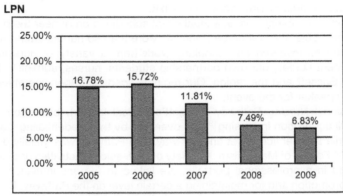

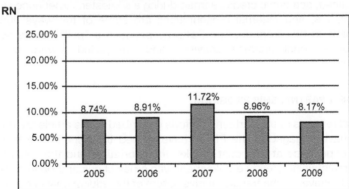

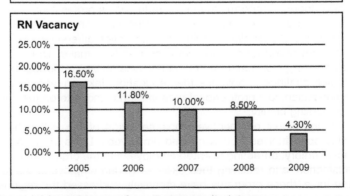

Fig. 3. Turnover and vacancy rates from Bassett Medical Center.

and serving to improve the structures, processes, and outcomes of patient care. Finally, these programs have provided nurses at the point of service with opportunities to expand their role and develop as practitioners through the nurse-preceptor or nursing faculty role, which allows the organization to retain the talents of clinically expert nurses while nurturing their further growth and development and affording them greater earning power and job satisfaction.

From the standpoint of the academic partners, these programs have increased the enrollment of nurses in these 2 local nursing schools and enhanced collaborative and strategic planning between nurse leaders in practice and academia. The programs have enhanced the practice environment and reduced the incidence of horizontal violence and negative interpersonal relationships in settings where students in all of our programs have clinical experiences. Indeed, students in the programs routinely remark on the positive reception that they get from staff nurses on the inpatient units at Bassett. These programs have primed the nursing faculty pipeline and encouraged clinically competent nurses at the point of service to engage in educating fellow professionals. Finally, these programs have encouraged the sharing of material and intellectual property, thus enhancing the teaching-learning experience for the benefit of students, faculty, nurses, and patients.

From a community perspective, rural residents who embark into careers in nursing have greater earning power that, in turn, positively affects the local economy.[5] Also, educational mobility programs that address the needs of the local learner and create career opportunities for career mobility are more likely to prevent or delay the phenomenon of rural to urban out-migration and the rural "brain drain" of highly skilled workers. In turn, a more educated health care workforce is likely to improve the community climate by providing positive role models to those young persons interested in a career in health care or nursing.[3,5,15] The partnerships directly or indirectly improve the economic health of Bassett and our local academic partners who are the major employers in this rural region.[5,16]

SUMMARY

There is nothing temporary about the challenges faced by rural hospitals in retaining and recruiting skillful nurses prepared to serve their patients. Bassett Medical Center has confronted this reality and established programs that aim to develop the local residents into a capable nursing staff. Academic agencies in the region participate in the programs, adding clear benefits as well as an added scholarly zest to the culture. The tuition assistance and the PNOP continue to be successful initiatives that support, educate, recruit, and retain talented individuals to work at Bassett Healthcare. The current pipeline to the schools is filled with pre-RNs who become attracted to the organizational and practice environments during summer internships. Residency programs are focused on newly hired nurses to socialize them into the professional environment and support their entry into practice and retain them. Faculty opportunities give seasoned Bassett nurses a different practice opportunity, which delights them and disseminates their expert practice. Magnet designation enrolls the organization in a high-performing community of other Magnet hospitals that focus on the care environment and the outcomes that make a difference for patients. We have seen the outcomes of these academic and service partnerships in nurses committed to advancing their education, serving in leadership positions, and acting as change agents. The success of these partnerships has helped nurse leaders at Bassett hold steady or decrease turnover rates and decrease RN vacancies while addressing the need for a more educated and engaged nursing workforce (**Fig. 3**).

REFERENCES

1. Dall TM, Cheu YJ, Seinfert RF, et al. The economic value of professional nursing. Med Care 2009;47(1):97–104. Available at: http://journals.lww.com/lww-medicalcare/pages/articleviewer.aspx?year=2009&issue=01000&article=00014&type=fulltext#. Accessed August 30, 2010.

2. Biviano MB, Tise S, Fritz M, et al. What is behind HRSA's projected supply, demand, and shortage of registered nurses? USDHHS, Bureau of Health Professions; 2004. Available at: ftp://ftp.hrsa.gov/bhpr/workforce/behindshortage.pdf. Accessed August 30, 2010.

3. Office of Rural Health and Primary Care, Minnesota DOH. Retaining rural nurses: midwestern summit on retaining and making best use of the older, more experienced rural registered nurse. 2007. Available at: http://www.health.state.mn.us/divs/orhpc/pubs/retainnurse.pdf. Accessed August 30, 2010.

4. Health Resources and Services Administration. Health professions shortage areas by state and county. Updated May 28, 2010. Available at: http://hpsafind.hrsa.gov/HPSASearch.aspx. Accessed August 30, 2010.

5. Barkley DL, Henry MS, Krozek C. Does human capital affect rural economic growth? Evidence from the South. Georgia: Clemson University Regional Development Research Laboratory; 2004. Research Report 03-2004-02. Available at: http://citeseerx.ist.psu.edu/viewdoc/summary?doi=10.1.1.152.3894. Accessed August 30, 2010.

6. USDA, Economic Research Services. Rural education at a glance. November 2003. Research Report No. 98. Available at: www.ers.usda.gov/publications/rdrr98/rdrr98_lowres.pdf. Accessed August 30, 2010.

7. Aiken LH, Clarke SP, Cheung RB, et al. Education levels of hospital nurses and surgical patient mortality. JAMA 2003;290(12):1617–23.

8. Stanton MW, Rutherford MK. Hospital nurse staffing and quality of care. Rockville (MD): AHRQ; 2004. Research in Action Issue No. 14. AHRQ Pub. No. 04-0029. Available at: http://www.ahrq.gov/research/nursestaffing/nursestaff.pdf. Accessed August 30, 2010.

9. U.S. Census Bureau, 2010 Census. NY State and County quick facts page. Updated August 16, 2010. Available at: http://quickfacts.census.gov/qfd/states/36000.html. Accessed August 30, 2010.

10. Brewer CS, Watkins R. Examining New York State nurses: a regional analysis of the 2004 National Sample Survey of Registered Nurses. 2004. Available at: http://www.ahec.buffalo.edu/resources/examining_2004_nys_nurses.pdf. Accessed August 30, 2010.

11. Healthcare Association of New York State (HANYS). HANYS workforce survey results for 2008: nursing and allied health professionals. 2008. Available at: http://www.hanys.org/workforce/reports/2008_workforce_survey_results.pdf. Accessed August 30, 2010.

12. NYS Dept of Education, Office of the Professions. Horizon issue: results of the September 2002 Survey of Registered Professional Nurses. 2003. Available at: http://www.op.nysed.gov/prof/nurse/nursing-survey-final-regents-report.htm. Accessed August 30, 2010.

13. Buerhaus PI, Auerbach DI, Staiger DO. The recent surge in nurse employment: causes and implications. Health Aff 2009;28(4):657–68. Available at: http://content.healthaffairs.org/cgi/content/abstract/hlthaff.28.4.w657. Accessed August 30, 2010.

14. NYSDOH. State and county health indicators (CHAI) for tracking public health priority areas. Updated January 2009. Available at: http://www.health.state.ny.us/prevention/prevention_agenda/indicator_map.htm. Accessed August 30, 2010.

15. NYS Department of Health. County health indicator profiles (CHIP) (2003–2007). Updated January 2009. Available at: http://www.health.state.ny.us/statistics/chip/index.htm. Accessed August 30, 2010.

16. Cornell University, Rural NY Initiative. NYS rural vision project: phase I summary report. 2006. Available at: http://devsoc.cals.cornell.edu/cals/devsoc/outreach/cardi/programs/indicators/rvp/upload/rvp-phase1report.pdf. Accessed August 30, 2010.

17. Beecraft PC, Kunzman L, Krozek C. RN internship – outcomes of a one-year pilot program. J Nurs Adm 2001;31(12):575–82.

18. Vermont Nurses in Partnership Page. Intern and preceptor development. Updated 2009. Available at: http://www.vnip.org/preceptor.html. Accessed August 30, 2010.

19. Benner P. From novice to expert: excellence and power in clinical nursing practice. Menlo Park (CA): Addison-Wesley; 1984.

20. Wolf G, Triolo P, Ponte PR. Magnet recognition program: the next generation. J Nurs Adm 2008;38(4):200–4.

21. Porter-O'Grady T, Hawkins M, Parker M. Whole systems shared governance: architecture for integration. Gathersburg (MD): Aspen Publishers; 1997.

22. StuderGroup Senior Nursing and Physician Leaders. The nurse leader handbook: the art and science of nurse leadership. Gulfstream (FL): Gulfstream Publishing; 2010.

23. Senge PM. The fifth discipline: the art and practice of the learning organization. New York: Doubleday/Currency; 1990.

24. PricewaterhouseCoopers, Health Research Institute. What works: healing the healthcare staffing shortages. 2007. Available at: http://www.pwc.com/us/en/healthcare/publications/what-works-healing-the-healthcare-staffing-shortage.jhtml. Accessed August 30, 2010.

Collaborative Research Partnerships in Support of Nursing Excellence

Karen Balakas, PhD, RN, CNE[a],*, Terry Bryant, MBA, BSN, RN, NE-BC[b],
Patricia Jamerson, PhD, RN, CRA, CCRP[b]

KEYWORDS

• Research • Partnerships • Nursing • Collaborate

Collaboration and the incorporation of research into nursing care delivery and the creation of new knowledge are characteristics of organizations that strive for excellence. The American Nurse Credentialing Center (ANCC) Magnet Recognition Program clearly indicates that to achieve magnet status an institution must demonstrate an environment that supports established and evolving programs of research and evidence-based practice.[1] As a free-standing, ANCC Magnet hospital within an academic medical center, St Louis Children's Hospital (SLCH) has an established history of conducting nursing research, establishing a culture to support evidence-based practice, and collaborating with community partners.

Research is an integral part of the mission and vision of SLCH. The nurses recognize the importance of providing evidence-based practice and their responsibility to contribute to the continued growth of nursing science through research. The hospital administration believes that questions posed by clinical nurses engaged in care delivery can contribute significantly to nursing's body of knowledge.

More than 2 decades ago, SLCH nursing leadership recognized the critical need for nursing research to enhance practice and develop policies and guidelines. The importance and value of research was demonstrated through initiatives to obtain a nurse researcher who could provide research leadership, develop an infrastructure supportive of research, provide research education, and obtain fiscal and administrative support for all steps in the research and dissemination process. However, resource limitations made it readily apparent that collaboration with academic partners within the medical center and beyond would be necessary to further develop and expand the research program.

The authors have nothing to disclose.
[a] Goldfarb School of Nursing at Barnes-Jewish College, 4483 Duncan Avenue, Mailstop 90-36-697, St Louis, MO 63110, USA
[b] St Louis Children's Hospital, One Children's Place, Suite PL-25, St Louis, MO 63110, USA
* Corresponding author.
E-mail address: KaBalakas@bjc.org

Nurs Clin N Am 46 (2011) 123–128
doi:10.1016/j.cnur.2010.10.006
0029-6465/11/$ – see front matter © 2011 Elsevier Inc. All rights reserved.

The idea of a partnership between a clinical and an academic institution is not a new concept; however, collaborating to enhance research within the clinical setting is a relatively novel concept. Partnerships between academic and clinical settings can result in numerous synergistic opportunities.[2] Recognizing this potential, SLCH continually seeks to develop research partnerships in a way that is mutually beneficial. The hospital offers clinical expertise and a venue for academicians to become engaged in an environment that values their scholarly contributions and academicians offer the hospital expertise in research and resources often limited in the clinical setting.

PARTNERING FOR BASIC ELEMENTS

From the onset of the research program, collaboration was necessary to provide for some of the most basic requirements for conducting research. One of these elements was the need for an Institutional Review Board (IRB) to ensure that proposed study procedures adhere to federal guidelines for the conduct of ethical research.[3] Because SLCH did not have its own IRB, the hospital negotiated with the Medical School IRB at Washington University (WU) in St Louis, a medical center partner, to provide this service. However, WU was not familiar with nursing research and some of the university policies were counterproductive (eg, the principal investigator must be doctorally prepared). Further negotiations resulted in changes in the IRB forms and processes to accommodate nursing research.

Unfamiliar with IRB review requirements, hospital staff also had difficulties obtaining timely IRB approval. To facilitate the review process, the nurse researcher and eventually other staff became IRB members to offer guidance and direction to hospital staff in the development of an IRB proposal. The review process was further enhanced by subjecting each study proposal to an administrative review by the nurse researcher and a scientific review by the hospital's Research Review Committee, before undergoing review by the WU IRB. In addition, WU made available to hospital staff the Collaborative Institutional Training Initiative's (CITI) human research subject's course and other workshops regarding the conduct of research offered to WU personnel.

Another basic requirement for research is the ability to search for and obtain current information in health care supplied by updated bibliographic and/or full-text databases.[4] Given the proximity of SLCH to the WU Medical Library, a collaborative agreement for library services also was negotiated with the university. The collaboration includes staffing of a satellite medical library within SLCH by a medical librarian and access to 33 databases including CINAHL Plus, MEDLINE, Health and Psychosocial Instruments (HAPI), and the Cochrane Library. The librarian is not only a valuable resource but also an active SLCH research committee member who also teaches classes for staff preparing to engage in research or evidence-based practice projects.

Conducting data analysis and interpreting statistical results can be a daunting task for many nurses and often becomes a barrier for engaging in research.[5] Although the SLCH research office performs data analysis, as the number of nurse investigators increased and studies became more complex, a need for more advanced programming and statistical support was realized. To meet this need, collaborative agreements were negotiated with medical center statisticians. Consultation with statisticians at the beginning of proposal development has resulted in increased staff understanding of the analysis plan, participation in data entry, and completion of studies.

COLLABORATION THROUGH COMMITTEE INVOLVEMENT

Another means to further develop a collaborative model between the hospital and academic partners was through the hospital's committee structure. Early in the development of the research program at SLCH, a nursing research committee was sanctioned to develop policies, procedures, and processes related to research, and to facilitate the conduct and dissemination of research. Because research is considered imperative to the academic role and nursing educators are expected to maintain strong links to the clinical field,[6] area nurse educators were invited to join the committee. It was believed that their involvement would help to expand the research knowledge base and to solicit research collaborators/mentors. Active involvement on the research committees also enabled nurse educators to understand more fully the organizational priorities for clinical research and to strengthen relationships with front-line staff who expressed an interest in research. Thus, this partnership also was reciprocally advantageous.

As the research program continued to grow, the Nursing Research Committee became multidisciplinary and evolved into a Research/Evidence-based Practice Advisory committee with 2 standing subcommittees: Research Review and Research Promotion. During this evolution, continued collaboration with nurse educators was deemed important to the success of the hospital-based research program. Academic partners helped to develop staff competency in evaluating proposed research and contributed to staff awareness of the importance of research for practice.

The Research Review committee was charged with performing a scientific review of each proposal, which includes evaluation of the overall design, theoretic/conceptual framework, methodology, data analysis plan, data monitoring plan, and budget. Because many of the staff nurses were not confident in their ability to independently perform a critical review of a research proposal, the nurse educators on the subcommittee were invaluable partners in the process. In turn, the nurse educators became more familiar with the hospital's research priorities, facilitating their own willingness to develop proposals and collaborate with staff on submissions.

The Research Promotion Committee was formed to identify educational needs of staff and develop strategies to promote research within the institution. Nurse educators also serve on this subcommittee, participating in the planning and delivery of workshops and the annual research and evidence-based practice conference, which is a venue for posters and oral presentations by both clinicians and educators.

COLLABORATION THROUGH NOVEL CLINICAL-ACADEMIC PROGRAMS

As the research program continued to grow, more creative ways to facilitate staff research were necessary. Given that the St Louis area is rich in the number of nursing schools, the research council identified ways to engage more nurse educators and their students. Two specialized programs were developed to enhance student and staff nurse knowledge and research skills and provide clinical research opportunities for educators.

Nursing Student Research Assistant Program

The Nursing Student Research Assistant Program (NS-RAP) was conceptualized as a way to garner for the hospital staff additional support to enroll subjects and collect and manage data. For the student nurses, NS-RAP was conceptualized as a means by which they could learn about and better appreciate the research process through active involvement.[7]

To participate, students completed an application process and negotiated with their faculty how the experience would be used to fulfill course requirements. After acceptance into the program, students completed the CITI human subjects training course, received instruction in how to obtain informed consent, and were trained in the use of the patient information system. Since its inception, 19 baccalaureate students and 25 graduate students have participated in the program and worked on several nursing studies. The program provided a meaningful learning experience for students and resulted in clinically relevant outcomes for the hospital.

Collaborative Faculty-Staff Research Grant Program

Another collaborative effort designed to develop the staff's research knowledge and contribute to nursing science is the collaborative faculty-staff research grant program. Funded by the hospital foundation, doctorally prepared nurse educators with pediatric/family research experience are invited to partner with hospital nurses to develop a proposal for a research project with significant potential to affect the clinical care of children. The Research Review Committee reviews the proposals. If funded, the nurse educator becomes a co-principal investigator with an SLCH nurse and is expected to mentor staff in the research process from research design to dissemination of the findings. Critical to the program is the involvement of clinicians from the beginning of all research activities so they are true partners in the project. Staff contribute to the proposal development, preparation of the IRB documents, data collection, data entry, analysis, and dissemination of findings. By their involvement in the process, staff are more apt to recognize the relevance and applicability of research findings and incorporate them into practice. The collaborative effort assures the nurse educator that the topic is important and directly applicable to clinical practice.

The program has been successful in generating research and engaging staff in all aspects of the process. Since its inception in 2007, the program has provided $56,590 to support 8 studies representing 11 faculty mentors from 5 schools and 21 clinicians (**Table 1** provides an overview of the studies to date). In the inaugural year of the program, 4 different studies with areas of focus on acute care and community-based research were supported. Year 2 expanded the program to include simulation and qualitative research. The program was expanded in 2009 to include allied health research faculty resulting in several multidisciplinary studies. At present, there are 4 studies in the review process for funding in 2010. Initial funding from the SLCH Foundation was granted for 1 year. Through collaboration with SLCH Foundation

Table 1
Collaborative faculty-staff grant program

Year	Study Title	Grant Award
2007	Effect of motivational interviewing on pediatric asthma management	$5650
2007	Creating opportunities for parent empowerment: a program for parents of chronically ill children	$8100
2007	Promotion of physical activity and prevention of obesity in children with asthma	$6500
2007	Family needs and family management styles of family caregivers of children with neurologic conditions during the neurorehabilitative phase	$9000
2008	High fidelity simulation: application for staff nurse education	$6700
2008	NICU nurses as NICU parents	$3440
2009	Medication adherence among adolescents undergoing a kidney transplant	$10,000
2009	DRINK study	$7200

Abbreviation: NICU, newborn intensive care unit.

leadership, grants were extended to 3 years (which was atypical for their processes), but reflected the complexity of conducting research.

Partnering for Simulation Research

Recent advances in simulation laboratories and training have provided additional forums for collaboration. Regional nursing programs have enhanced education with the addition of simulation centers and there is considerable research to support the use of simulation for education. However, there is little research to date that explores the use of simulation for staff education in the clinical setting. In 2009, SLCH opened the Saigh Pediatric Simulation Center and academic partners assisted the hospital's simulation clinical education specialist with scenario development strategies and debriefing techniques. The partnerships in simulation have resulted in several collaborative research projects with a variety of focus. Studies have included the use of simulation for multidisciplinary team training, nursing recognition of the deteriorating patient, nursing response to malignant hyperthermia for the surgical patient, and safety and cognitive functioning in transport team nurses working extended shifts.

Collaborative Joint Research Appointment

Yet another collaborative venture was the Collaborative Joint Research Appointment. While the hospital searched for another nurse researcher, the Goldfarb College of Nursing within the medical center concurrently was refocusing more time for faculty scholarly endeavors and actively sought opportunities to expand relationships with clinical facilities. As a result, negotiations ensued between SLCH and the Goldfarb College of Nursing to create a joint appointment between the college and the hospital. In addition to the academic qualifications, it was essential that the nurse researcher chosen for the joint position possess the ability to generate enthusiasm for bedside nursing research and have a foundation in the application of evidence-based practice in a clinical setting. Within 5 months, negotiations were complete and the faculty nurse researcher was available to the staff.

Through this partnership, the research department gained additional resources to assist nursing staff in study design, identification of funding opportunities, preparation of proposals for internal and external review, grant proposal preparation, tool identification or development, data management and analysis, and dissemination of results. The faculty nurse researcher also co-chairs the Research/Evidence-based Practice Advisory committee, teaches research and evidence-based practice workshops, and serves on several hospital committees to promote scholarship and support the Magnet journey.

COLLABORATION GENERATES BENEFITS

Collaborating with academic partners provides measurable and nonmeasurable benefits for both parties. Through the collaborative efforts previously described, research has been successfully incorporated into hospital culture and many research projects, publications, and presentations have ensued. But some of the less objective outcomes are the appreciation of the staff for research and evidence-based practice and respect for the nurse educators with whom they have partnered to create the research environment at SLCH and conduct research.

There have also been benefits for the nurse educators. Development of a collaborative model increases faculty knowledge of the complexities of health care and provides opportunities for research. Faculty are encouraged and supported to use their research skills in a clinical setting and collaboration with practitioners who are better placed to identify researchable questions have resulted in studies that are clinically meaningful and have the potential to change practice. As with a true collaborative model, the value of mutual interdependency is recognized and honored by both clinicians and academicians.[8]

SUMMARY

Promoting research and evidence-based practice are foundational to enhancing the body of nursing knowledge and the continued development and enrichment of nurses. Partnering with academic colleagues is an effective way to increase the number of staff nurses participating in research projects that would not have been possible with existing resources. In addition, the number of poster presentations, oral presentations, and publications has continued to increase, adding to the overall knowledge of nursing.

REFERENCES

1. American Nurses Credentialing Center. Application manual: magnet recognition program. Silver Springs (MD): American Nurses Credentialing Center; 2008. p. 50.
2. Newhouse RP. Collaborative synergy: practice and academic partnerships in evidence-based practice. J Nurs Adm 2007;37(3):105–8.
3. Polit DF, Beck CT. Essentials of nursing research: appraising evidence for nursing practice. 7th edition. Philadelphia: Lippincott Williams & Wilkins; 2010. p. 132–3.
4. Fineout-Overhold E, Stillwell SB, Williamson KM, et al. Teaching evidence-based practice in academic settings. In: Melnyk BM, Fineout-Overholt E, editors. Evidence-based practice in nursing & healthcare: a guide to best practice. 2nd edition. Philadelphia: Lippincott Williams & Wilkins; 2011. p. 306–7.
5. Albert NM, Siedlecki SL. Developing and implementing a nursing research team in a clinical setting. J Nurs Adm 2008;38(2):90–6.
6. Happell B. Clinical-academic partnerships research: converting the rhetoric into reality. Int J Psychiatr Nurs Res 2005;11(1):1218–26.
7. Jamerson PA, Fish AF, Frandsen G. Nursing student research assistant program: a strategy to enhance nursing research capacity building in a Magnet status pediatric hospital. Appl Nurs Res 2009. DOI: 10.1016/j.apnr.2009.08.004.
8. Springer PJ, Corbett C, Davis N. Enhancing evidence-based practice through collaboration. J Nurs Adm 2006;36(11):534–7.

Shaping Future Nurse Leaders Through Shared Governance

Joan Ellis Beglinger, RN, MSN, MBA[a],*, Barbara Hauge, RN, BSN[b],
Sheryl Krause, RN, MS, CEN, ACNS-BC[c], Laura Ziebarth, RN, MSN[d]

KEYWORDS

• Shared governance • Nursing leadership • Leaders

Each year, the nursing literature is rich with articles about the professional practice model most commonly known as shared governance. The American Nurses Credentialing Center Magnet Recognition Program emphasis on structural empowerment has served to intensify interest in this model. Areas of focus are diverse and include research studies to measure impact and effectiveness, journeys taken and insights gained, and examples of various models and their perceived benefits. Common themes include strengthening professional practice, driving improved clinical outcomes, enhancing professional nurse engagement, and advancing professional development.[1–5] Strikingly absent from the professional literature is evidence that shared governance is an ideal vehicle for the development of future nurse leaders. The purpose of this article is to begin to close that gap—to share the experience of one 440-bed tertiary acute care hospital and how its 18-year journey to a mature shared governance model has produced five unit directors and three clinical nurse specialists from the ranks of former council chairs.

BACKGROUND

In 1991, the nursing organization of St Mary's Hospital in Madison, Wisconsin, began to transform itself from a traditional hierarchy to a model of shared governance. The members of the organization recognized the need to restructure, to enable themselves to function as a professional discipline within the context of the hospital and assume ownership for the work of nursing. With assistance and guidance from Tim Porter-O'Grady, DM, EdD, APRN, FAAN, as a consultant regarding shared governance, a structure was implemented, extensive development ensued, and the journey was

[a] Patient Care Services, St Mary's Hospital, 700 South Park Street, Madison, WI 53715, USA
[b] Medical/Surgical, St Mary's Hospital, 700 South Park Street, Madison, WI 53715, USA
[c] Emergency Services, St Mary's Hospital, 700 South Park Street, Madison, WI 53715, USA
[d] NICU and Pediatrics, St Mary's Hospital, 700 South Park Street, Madison, WI 53715, USA
* Corresponding author.
E-mail address: Joan_Beglinger@ssmhc.com

Nurs Clin N Am 46 (2011) 129–135
doi:10.1016/j.cnur.2010.10.003
0029-6465/11/$ – see front matter © 2011 Elsevier Inc. All rights reserved.

nursing.theclinics.com

undertaken. In 2002, St Mary's achieved the 50th Magnet designation by the American Nurses Credentialing Center. That same year, St Mary's Hospital, as a member of SSM Health Care, became the first nursing organization in the country to become both Magnet recognized and a recipient of the Malcolm Baldrige National Quality Award. In addition, SSM Health Care was the first health care organization in the country to be awarded the coveted Baldrige award. For several years, St Mary's remained the only Magnet recognized recipient of the Baldrige award in the nation. In 2006, St Mary's was redesignated as a Magnet organization and in 2010 will pursue its second redesignation.

Throughout 18 years of experience in the shared governance journey, many cycles of improvement have taken place. Enhancements to the strategic planning process, improved communication linkages, and more effective approaches to professional development are but a few examples of the progress that has been made. Despite significant, deliberate attention that has been paid to continuously improving the structure, process, and outcomes, it was only in hindsight that it became clear that leadership development has been a definite, if not planned, outcome of shared governance.

The benefits of developing an organization's future leaders from within have been promoted by some of the truly exemplary organizations of our time. The Mayo Clinic has long attributed sustained organizational excellence to the development of leaders who understand the culture and are committed to its values and to a leadership approach that has proved effective.[6] Although there are compelling reasons to recruit some future leaders from outside an organization, including a need to make significant change or to introduce unique expertise into the team, there is a widespread belief that developing leadership talent from within serves to strengthen an enterprise and thus the workforce in multiple dimensions.

SHARED GOVERNANCE'S CONTRIBUTION TO LEADERSHIP DEVELOPMENT

The collective insights of those within St Mary's who have progressed through clinical leadership positions within shared governance to unit director and clinical nurse specialist roles, coupled with the reflections of the organization's nurse executive, have produced our contemporary understanding of the experiences within shared governance that shape future leaders. These insights will undoubtedly change and grow as others contribute to our knowledge with their experiences in the future.

Getting Noticed and Nudged

Traditional hierarchies create barriers between the point of service and those who serve in administrative roles. Hierarchies are often comprised of multiple layers of management and it is common in these structures for senior leaders to operate somewhat distant from, and in isolation from, those who do the work of the organization.[7] Discovering talent and seeing the potential that resides within individuals whose work is far removed from the administrative suite is impossible if executives' lives do not intersect with the point of care. Shared governance, by definition, supports a flat organizational structure. Professionals with clinical roles find themselves shoulder to shoulder with professionals with administrative roles during the course of their work. The design of the framework is a partnership where decision making is shared. The visibility that is afforded the clinical professional in this model is extensive and the opportunity to be noticed and nudged as an employee is a regular occurrence. As administrators and clinical professionals come to know one another as colleagues, conversations evolve and mentoring occurs both on a formal and informal basis.

A comment as seemingly casual as an executive's observation about a clinician's future potential can inspire confidence and dreams that might not have otherwise been conceived. In the words of a now successful clinical nurse specialist, "It was critical to my career path that those I looked up to and respected took the time to reinforce the behaviors they wanted me to continue and gave me honest feedback about what I might consider doing differently."

Developing an Understanding of the Big Picture

The development of a systems point of view and an appreciation of the big picture perspective further position clinical nurse leaders within a shared governance system to take their next step on the leadership continuum.

Shared governance clinical nurse leaders at St Mary's are considered part of the official leadership structure. As such, they are included in activities that expose them to information and experiences that would be otherwise invisible to them. The chair of the Nursing Coordinating Council, as an example, is considered the chief of the nursing organization and is included in the same way as the chief of the medical staff in hospital operations. The chair officially represents nursing during such significant events as Joint Commission surveys, Magnet site visits, and Malcolm Baldrige site visits, to name a few. The chair is an active member of the hospital strategic planning committee and the budget committee. In these roles she brings the important clinical nursing perspective to deliberations and is also exposed, for the first time, to some of the major processes used in the leadership of the hospital.

All of the clinical chairs of shared governance are included in an annual rollout of the regional strategic plan, are appointed to clinically focused interdisciplinary committees, and are included in communications to hospital leadership that, in traditional organizations, would be limited to the line management structure. The opportunities for the clinical nurse leaders of shared governance to be exposed to the broader functioning of the hospital create the catalyst for them to think about their own futures in expanded terms. Possibilities take on depth and meaning beyond the boundaries of their home unit.

In addition to developing an expanded understanding of the hospital system in which they practice, the clinical nurse leaders of the shared governance structure report new and more comprehensive thinking about the profession of nursing itself. In the words of a former chair who went on to assume the role of clinical nurse specialist, "Leadership of a shared governance council informed my thinking about my obligation to further the profession of Nursing."

The experience of leading a council in shared governance has proved instrumental in expanding understanding of the system of care as well as the profession of nursing. Each role has proved to serve as a stimulus to further thoughts about future roles in permanent leadership roles and provides a framework to sort through the decision-making process that pushes a nurse toward management or pulls her to an advanced practice role.

Results Orientation

The development of a results orientation is another key contribution of the experience of shared governance leadership. All leaders are fundamentally concerned with producing results. Either facilitating the system of care in a management role or advancing the practice of the profession through a clinical role, the focus on desired outcomes and the strategies to achieve them are common threads.

Nurses leading the councils in a shared governance model are integrally involved in the development of the strategic plan for nursing (which has evolved into the outcomes management plan at St Mary's in recognition of the primary obligation to achieve outcomes). The plan is aligned with the strategic priorities of the entire health system, our region, and our hospital, and addresses the specific role of nursing in achieving the broader plan. The work of the year is focused around the strategic priorities. Specific plans are developed, metrics defined and monitored, and progress tracked. Nurse leaders become proficient in thinking of their work in terms of the outcomes produced.

Even though, the process of becoming a manager or a leader may not yet be fully developed or described; it seems certain that an orientation toward outcomes is one of the characteristics to emerge in those who effectively lead and that experience in leadership in our shared governance structure supports this competency.

Skill Acquisition

The opportunity for extensive skill acquisition as the chair of a shared governance council provides tremendous preparation for future leadership roles. Development occurs through both formal and experiential learning and can range from technical to conceptual. Examples are included for their instructive value but are by no means exhaustive.

- Interpersonal skill development—In the role of council chair, it has been common for nurses to find themselves delivering presentations before groups of people. Formal presentations of the nursing organization's work at such noteworthy gatherings as the American College of Healthcare Executives annual congress or the American Organization of Nurse Executives annual conference have been highlights for the nurses who participated. Annual consultations on our shared governance success, hosted by our nursing organization, and a biannual national conference, hosted five times over a decade by our organization, provided venues for our nurses to develop skill at presenting their work. These avenues, coupled with the less formal daily interactions with many people throughout the organization, provide tremendous opportunity to observe those who are more experienced in public presentation skills and to practice and learn to communicate effectively in this regard. Poise and confidence are developed through these experiences and add to individuals' growing list of attributes that position them to compete for a future leadership role.
- Organizational skill development—The art of facilitating group work is learned behavior. Preparing an agenda, managing time, managing group dynamics, and ensuring the achievement of desired outcomes all require skill acquisition and practice. Preparation to assume the leadership of a council includes formal, didactic sessions focused on skill building in these areas. Productive meetings are essential to generating results.
- Computer skill development—Nurses come to leadership roles in shared governance with varied experience and expertise in working with computer technology. Basic tools, such as e-mail and PowerPoint, may be new to them. Many formal educational programs as well as one-on-one tutoring opportunities are available to ensure that nurse leaders are able to leverage the vast technology of our system in fulfilling their roles.
- Acquisition of continuous quality improvement (CQI) tools and techniques—In the early 1990s, SSM Health Care began a journey of continuous quality

improvement. This pursuit involved fundamental principles of improvement, including:

Patients and other customers are our first priority
All work is part of a process
Quality is achieved through people
Decisions should be based on facts
Quality requires continuous improvement.

A curriculum was developed and made available throughout the SSM Health System to facilitate the organization's learning and application of continuous improvement methodology. Nursing council chairs were among the priority candidates for these learning opportunities. Although the evolution of SSM Health Care has resulted in changes in our understanding of, and approach to, CQI methodology, shared governance leaders remain actively engaged in the educational process, including participation in the development and piloting of new courses.

The benefits of the skills acquired through service as a clinical nurse leader within shared governance extend far beyond their usefulness in preparing future nurse leaders. Time and again, unit directors report that on returning to practice after tenure as a council chair, nurses demonstrate tremendous growth in their approach to patient care and to the challenges that present at the unit level.

NEXT STEPS

Growing awareness that leadership in shared governance is powerful in the development of future nurse leaders has prompted consideration of the next steps for our organization. Three areas of focus have been identified as we strive to continually strengthen and improve ourselves. They are the implementation of whole system shared decision making (WSSDM), a formalized approach to succession planning, and the development of a core curriculum for leaders and members of shared governance and WSSDM councils that will include the articulation and measurement of essential competencies.

WSSDM

The clear success of the shared governance model in nursing over many years prompted the administrative team to commit to this organizational structure for the entire hospital. In 2008, Dr Porter O'Grady was again engaged, an interdisciplinary steering team was formed, and a comprehensive planning process was undertaken. In the fall of 2010, the first councils were formed and the WSSDM structure was launched. It is anticipated that the transition from nursing to whole system will be every bit as noisy and painful as the transition of nursing from hierarchy to shared governance. Tremendous new learning will be required of every manager and of every employee. Experience has taught that sustained cultural changes of this magnitude are a multiyear process. We eagerly anticipate the emergence of new leaders from every part of the organization and are firmly committed to our belief that leveraging the talent of the organization will be our most significant competitive advantage.

Nursing has played a prominent role in planning for the transition to WSSDM. A former chair of the Nursing Coordinating Council and a director, who was the former chair of the Management Council, have served on the steering team. The nurse executive was a frequent consultant to the steering team as they encountered questions or obstacles during the transition. There has been a deliberate and successful attempt to balance capitalizing on nursing's expertise and experience in the development of

WSSDM while avoiding the perception that "the nursing way" is overtaking the organization. Nurses who are experienced in shared governance will serve on each WSSDM council in the future as a means of supporting the transition.

Succession Planning

The outcomes management plan for nursing for 2010 includes the development and implementation of a succession planning process for nurses who wish to pursue clinical and managerial leadership roles. In our conversations as a management team, we have concluded that if we do not have at least one outstanding candidate to succeed the director on each unit, we have not fulfilled our accountability to develop people. Similarly, it is a goal of our nursing organization to have enough enthusiastic, highly qualified candidates for each open position in our council or structure so that elections are required each year to provide enough opportunities for those who are interested. Advanced practice nurses should also emerge from within our ranks to meet our needs as they develop through the council or structure.

Development of the succession process is in its early stages. A variety of strategies are being developed for management succession, including forums in which nurses can learn about the work of management, programs where nurses can hear about the experiences of nurses who have progressed from clinical practitioner to director, and a formal mentoring process for nurses who have identified that management is a career goal, which will include structured exposure to various facets of the management role. On the clinical side, the process will include mechanisms for nurses to learn more about leadership on councils and the roles of advanced practitioners, with structured learning opportunities related to both.

Core Curriculum for Leadership Development

The final component in our plan for next steps is the development of a robust, structured core curriculum for the development of leaders within the organization. Clearly defined leadership competencies, structured educational experiences, and measurement of the effectiveness of the teaching and learning are all considered essential elements that we currently lack. The Coordinating Council is working closely with the organization's CQI director and the manager of organizational development to construct a well thought-out approach that will meet the needs of emerging leaders in the years to come. The availability of a systematic approach to the acquisition and transfer of leadership knowledge and skills will close a significant gap that currently exists within our organization.

SUMMARY

The progression of five professional nurses from shared governance council chairs to unit director positions and the progression of three nurses from shared governance council chairs to clinical nurse specialist roles in an 18-year period provide compelling evidence of the impact shared governance has provided in the development of future nurse leaders in our organization. The collective wisdom of those who have lived this experience suggests that the opportunities that are inherent in these clinical nurse leadership roles make this a logical progression. The opportunities include getting noticed and nudged, developing an understanding of the big picture, developing a results orientation, and substantial skill acquisition. More study is required to enable nursing to leverage shared governance as a vehicle for leadership development as we support the career progression of nurse leaders in the future.

REFERENCES

1. Church JA, Baker P, Berry DM. Shared governance: a journey with continual mile markers. Nurs Manage 2008;39:35–40.
2. Bogue RJ, Joseph ML, Sieloff CL. Shared governance as vertical alignment of nursing group power and nurse practice council effectiveness. J Nurs Manag 2009;17:4–14.
3. Malleo C, Fusilero J. Shared governance: withstanding the test of time. Nurse Leader 2009;32–6.
4. Watters S. Shared leadership taking flight. J Nurs Admin 2009;39(1):26–9.
5. Kramer M, Schmalenber C, Maguire P, et al. Walk the talk: promoting control of nursing practice and a patient-centered culture. Crit Care Nurse 2009;29(3): 77–93.
6. Seltman KD, Berry LL. Enduring leadership: lessons from the mayo clinic. Leader Leader 2009;8–12.
7. Hammett P. The paradox of gifted leadership: developing the generation of leaders. Ind Commerc Train 2008;40(1):3–9.

Index

Note: Page numbers of article titles are in **boldface** type.

Moving?

Make sure your subscription moves with you!

To notify us of your new address, find your **Clinics Account Number** (located on your mailing label above your name), and contact customer service at:

Email: journalscustomerservice-usa@elsevier.com

800-654-2452 (subscribers in the U.S. & Canada)
314-447-8871 (subscribers outside of the U.S. & Canada)

Fax number: 314-447-8029

Elsevier Health Sciences Division
Subscription Customer Service
3251 Riverport Lane
Maryland Heights, MO 63043

Printed and bound by CPI Group (UK) Ltd, Croydon, CR0 4YY

03/10/2024

01040445-0015